NATIVE AMERICAN RESOURCES SERIES

1. *Handbook of the American Frontier: Four Centuries of Indian–White Relationships*, by J. Norman Heard
   Volume I: *Southeastern Woodlands.* 1987.
   Volume II: *Northeastern Woodlands.* 1990.
   Volume III: *The Great Plains.* 1993.
   Volume IV: *The Far West.* 1997.
   Volume V: *Chronology, Bibliography, Index.* 1998.
2. *Oliver La Farge and the American Indian*, by Robert A. Hecht. 1991.
3. *Native American Resurgence and Renewal: A Reader and a Bibliography*, by Robert N. Wells, Jr. 1994.
4. *The Navajo as Seen by the Franciscans, 1898–1921: A Sourcebook*, edited by Howard M. Bahr. 2004.
5. *Forgotten Voices: Death Records of the Yakama, 1888–1964*, by Clifford E. Trafzer and Robert R. McCoy. 2009.

FORGOTTEN VOICES

Death Records of the Yakama, 1888–1964

Clifford E. Trafzer
Robert R. McCoy

Native American Resources, No. 5

THE SCARECROW PRESS, INC.
Lanham, Maryland • Toronto • Plymouth, UK
2009

SCARECROW PRESS, INC.

Published in the United States of America
by Scarecrow Press, Inc.
A wholly owned subsidiary of
The Rowman & Littlefield Publishing Group, Inc.
4501 Forbes Boulevard, Suite 200, Lanham, Maryland 20706
www.scarecrowpress.com

Estover Road
Plymouth PL6 7PY
United Kingdom

British Library Cataloguing in Publication Information Available

Library of Congress Cataloging-in-Publication Data

Trafzer, Clifford E.
Forgotten voices : death records of the Yakama, 1888–1964 / Clifford E. Trafzer, Robert R. McCoy.
p. cm. — (Native American resources ; no. 5)
Includes bibliographical references.
ISBN-13: 978-0-8108-6647-8 (cloth : alk. paper)
ISBN-10: 0-8108-6647-1 (cloth : alk. paper)
ISBN-13: 978-0-8108-6648-5 (eBook)
ISBN-10: 0-8108-6648-X (eBook)
1. Yakama Indians—Mortality—Statistics. 2. Yakama Indians—Diseases—Statistics. 3. Yakama Indians—Health and hygiene—Statistics. 4. Yakama Indian Reservation (Wash.)—Statistics, Medical. 5. Yakama Indian Reservation (Wash.)—Statistics, Vital. I. McCoy, Robert R. (Robert Ross), 1962– II. Title.
E99.Y2T74 2009
614.4'2797089974127—dc22

2008043088

∞™ The paper used in this publication meets the minimum requirements of American National Standard for Information Sciences—Permanence of Paper for Printed Library Materials, ANSI/NISO Z39.48-1992.

Manufactured in the United States of America.

To the descendents of these families:

Kamiakin, Owhi, Teias, Quetalakin, Peopeo Kownot,
Tomeo, Hemene Moxmox, Hemene Kawan, Hahtalekin,
Husishusis Kute, Hinmahtooyahlatkekht

Contents

Series Editor's Foreword

As this book goes to press, the U.S. Senate has overwhelmingly passed a bill to dramatically increase federal spending on Native American health care. The legislation authorizes an appropriation of $35 billion during the next decade for the construction and modernization of hospitals and clinics throughout the nation, and for the augmentation of medical staffs, upgrading of equipment, and the expansion of services. New programs will likewise coordinate tribal access to Medicare and Medicaid, and remove some of the bureaucratic barriers that have prevented American Indians from seeking help to which they are already legally entitled. In speaking for passage of this bill, Senator Byron Dorgan, chairman of the Senate Committee on Indian Affairs, listed numerous examples of the historical failures of the Indian Health Service and the long-term consequences on native peoples. He labeled this effort as a first step toward repairing a system that is underfunded and inefficient. Senate Majority Leader Harry Reid echoed the sentiment and labeled Indian health care as "some of the least-adequate health care in America." The bill also includes a provision sponsored by Senator Sam Brownback that apologizes to Native Americans for two centuries of government mistreatment.

Despite passage of a similar bill in the House Natural Resources Committee and House Energy and Commerce Subcommittee, the potential law has a long way to go before attaining approval in amended form. President George W. Bush has already demanded the deletion of some provisions within the legislation and the Senate has agreed to remove these requirements to avoid a White

House veto. Much of the debate centers on funding this large-scale program and keeping it within the anticipated federal budget levels during the next ten years.

The facts are undeniable that the Indian Health Service has failed to live up to expectations since its founding in 1955. Statistics speak to some of that reality. Native Americans evidence twice the national average of sudden infant death syndrome, a tuberculosis rate 453 percent higher than the American average, chronic liver disease and cirrhosis at approximately 500 percent higher than the national average, and an alcohol-related death rate among youths that is 17 times higher than for all other races in the national population.

Despite great progress in lowering the incidents of "infectious diseases" that afflicted early- to mid-20th-century American Indian populations, the new "behavior-related diseases" pose the greatest threat today. Especially noteworthy are dietary problems, tobacco abuse, alcoholism, drug abuse, hypertension, obesity, cardiovascular disease, and diabetes. Some tribal governments have been able to enter into contract agreements with the Indian Health Service and other government agencies so that they can oversee their own health care facilities and even set policies for them. Other tribal governments and urban Indian centers have attracted outside sources of revenue to supplement their delivery programs. And in many cases, traditional medicine men and healers now work within medical facilities to help address holistic approaches to recovery.

Doctors Clifford Trafzer of the University of California at Riverside and Robert McCoy of Washington State University have now provided readers and researchers with a unique collection of material that allows for a case-study approach to many of these medical problems. By focusing upon the Yakama of the Pacific Northwest during the twentieth century, they have identified the evolution of different health conditions over the decades. Furthermore, they have analyzed how cultural changes have altered patterns of tribal life, and, in turn, have defined both improving and worsening health care conditions. Trafzer's and McCoy's work demonstrates how meticulous research in death records can illuminate much about the evolution of a people and can speak to today's ambiguous patterns in health care delivery. Hopefully, their efforts will spur other researchers from a host of academic disciplines to delve into similar records of other tribal peoples, and provide solid evidence for formulating wiser policies in today's inefficient and sometimes misguided health care system.

Specific materials discussed in this foreword are taken from two sources: "Senate Approves Bill on Indian Health Care," *Omaha World Herald* (February 27, 2008); and The Harvard Project on American Indian Economic Development, *The State of the Native Nations: Conditions under U.S. Policies of Self-Determination* (New York: Oxford University Press, 2008): 219–33.

—Michael Tate, professor of history and Native American studies,
University of Nebraska at Omaha

Preface

In October 2006, the Plateau Indian Center of Washington State University hosted an annual conference that focused on the survival of the descendants of Palouse Indians. Some people of Palouse Indian descent live on the Yakama Reservation, while others live on the Warm Springs, Colville, Umatilla, Nez Perce, and other Northwestern Indian reservations. The people came together with scholars interested in Plateau Indian studies, and conference participants spent three days in several sessions discussing and analyzing the historical and cultural changes that had resulted in the great diaspora of Palouse people to many different reservations. The conference began in a traditional manner with Wendell Jim, director of education for the Warm Springs Tribe of Oregon, inviting elders to come forward to begin the gathering through song and prayer.

Tribal elders from many different Indian reservations came forward to share their culture, some of them moving slowly in wheelchairs. The men stood in the background and the women stepped forward. A singer began the first of many songs, singing a prayer that brought the power to bear on that time and place. As the people sang, many of us thought of the old ones. They came to our minds and we remembered them. They had shown us the way in our lives and work. In the 1970s and 1980s, tribal elders and teachers had instructed the authors about the history of the people, and they had told us of their parents, grandparents, friends, and kin. We had learned through oral histories and narratives about the elders and their lives during the wars of the 19th century and their confinements onto reservations. Although most of the elders we had known in the decades past have passed over, their children and grandchildren continued their work and taught us more. These contemporary Indian people had come from a hearty stock. They were the descendents of people who had survived the invasion of their land, the forced takeover of many aspects of their lives. At the conference, Indians and non-Indians came together to discuss the survival of the people, their culture, and their languages. As they sang their sacred songs, the tribal people provided testimonials to the spiritual strength and vitality of the people. Their religious convictions and their spiritual ways had bound the people together in the past and had carried them into the future. The singers were descendents of survivors, and like their own elders, they refused to surrender the spiritual foundations of the people, the unseen power that had kept the people together for generations.

This work is the result of over 25 years of research in the National Archives and on the reservations of the Pacific Northwest. The major focus of this work is the statistical data derived from the death certificates of American Indian people from many different Indian tribes that the government had forced onto the Yakama Indian Reservation. It is also a result of some oral histories conducted in the 1970s and 1980s, as well as the use of excellent secondary and primary sources. The authors view the statistics found in this volume to be the voices of the dead, and we feel that the statistical voices are alive with meaning. For us, the people speak through their deaths, telling us about life and death on one reservation during the turbulent transitional era of American history when the government attempted to destroy Indian people, their cultures, languages, and religions. The data speak in many ways, and we have provided some of our interpretations in the introduction of this work. This is not the first study based on the statistics taken from the death certificates of the Yakama Indian Reservation. In 1997, Clifford Trafzer published a social and medical history, *Death Stalks the Yakama*. He used the statistics found in this study, and with Rob McCoy, has continued the research on Yakama mortality and survival. McCoy and Trafzer have expanded the research through this study, offering other original sources for future scholarly use. They are also focusing future research on accidents, suicides, and murders on the Yakama Reservation, so these data are not included in the present study. The work offers nearly all of the statistics dealing with mortality of Yakama people from 1888 to 1964, and we encourage scholars, buffs, and members of the Indian communities of the Northwest to use our data. We hope that our work will encourage others to expand the Yakama story and compare these statistics with future data sets created by others.

We feel that the data found in this volume support the conclusion that the United States set out to destroy Yakama people and their culture through war, removal, and the reservation system. The government did not support Yakama people minimally, not even to the extent promised in the Yakama

Treaty of 1855. Using the definition of genocide offered by the United Nations in 1948, we have concluded that the government committed several acts whose "intent [was] to destroy, in whole or in part, a national, ethnical, racial or religious group."[1] The government committed genocide through killings, causing bodily and mental harm, inflicting conditions calculated to bring about the physical destruction of the people, imposing measures intended to prevent births, and forcibly transferring children to other groups such as Christian missionaries and boarding school superintendents.

Scholars, buffs, and citizens of the United States may wish to disagree with our interpretation about genocide, but for us, mortality statistics from the reservation era demonstrate the ways in which the Office of Indian Affairs ignored the large number of deaths on the reservation and pushed its agenda to assimilate Indians without regard to their ultimate survival as people. The government's actions and/or inactions supported the destruction of Yakama people, causing serious harm to the health and well-being of men, women, and children. These deaths testify to the fact that the government did not provide Yakama people with health care, hospitals, nutritious food, or public health education so they could isolate patients and successfully fight bacteria and viruses through sanitation efforts. The government failed in its obligations and the people died as a result. The nation turned its back on Yakama people who suffered a domestic genocide from which the people are still attempting to overcome—a genocide denied by many but not the Indian people who suffered the consequences of government policies.

We are grateful to many people for helping us with this research and publication. The Indian people of the Northwest have been very gracious with their time and expertise, and we thank Mary Jim, Emily Peone, Andrew George, Tom Estama, Ron Pond, Bobby Conners, Carrie Jim, Albert Redstar Andrews, Attwice Kamiakun, Josiah Pinkham, Gordon Fisher, and Tanya Tomeo. We offer a special thanks to Richard D. Scheuerman, Michelle Raheja, Rebecca Kugel, and Orlan Svingen, our friends and colleagues who have encouraged us with this work. Moreover, we thank a number of scholars who have contributed to our work either through their own research, editing, encouragement, or letters, including Eugene Hunn, Robert Boyd, Christie Firtha, Abdel Omran, Neal Hickman, Helen Schuster, William Medina, and John Weeks. We extend our appreciation for their assistance to Joyce Justice, formerly of the National Archives, Pacific Northwest Region, Melissa Conway of Special Collections at the University of California, Riverside, and Colleen Veomett of the Yakama Tribal Library. Dean Stephen Cullenberg of the University of California, Riverside, and Patrick King of Washington State University have also supported our research in this project, and we respectfully thank them for their continued support of our academic work. We also thank Michael Tate and Jack Marken, editors of the Native American Bibliography and Resource Series of Scarecrow Press, who encouraged us to research this work. We extend our greatest gratitude to Lee Ann and Julie as well as our children, all of whom gave us precious time to work. Finally, we offer our condolences to the families of the Yakama people who lost so many loved ones. We hope that our work brings voice to those who have passed on, those who still play a role in the lives of contemporary people and this academic work.

Note

1. See *Convention on the Prevention and Punishment of the Crime of Genocide*, adopted by Resolution 260 (III) A of the United Nations General Assembly on 9 December 1948: www.hrweb.org/legal/genocide.html.

Introduction

DEATH IS THE COMMON DENOMINATOR for all human beings. In the last two decades, more and more scholars have focused on the nature and dimensions of disease and death among native peoples in the Western hemisphere. While recognizing the destruction of initial epidemics and their impact on political, economic, social, and cultural institutions, scholars often stopped their narratives with the completion of European or Anglo-American conquest and the confiscation of Indian territories by empires or nation states. It is not our belief that this was a conscious silencing of discussions of Native American death after conquest or relegation to reservations. Instead, it seems that the more dramatic deaths, the enormous loss of life associated with the onset of diseases unknown in the Americas, caught the attention of both scholars and the public alike. Until recently, studies of death and its causes during the reservation period of the late nineteenth and early twentieth centuries seemed less interesting or at least not as relevant.

When discussing death and the history of Native Americans during the late nineteenth and early twentieth centuries, it is imperative to analyze and deconstruct the powerful myth of the disappearing Indian. Most narratives created by Anglo-Americans during this period mentioned the "inevitable" demise of Native Americans. For Anglo-Americans, death and assimilation worked together to destroy cultures that they deemed inferior, or at the very least incapable of progress and civilization. The myth served Anglo-Americans well and not only justified military conquest and theft of native lands, but also served as an explanation for the continued death of Indians confined to reservations. In essence, the myth of the disappearing Indian was a balm for the conscience of Anglo-Americans, a cure-all explanation for the perceived condition of Native Americans both before and after their imprisonment on reservations.

In the role of the disappearing or vanishing Indian, Native Americans were, according to the myth, incapable of resisting the dual onslaughts of Anglo-American civilization and disease. This passivity fit nicely into preconceived ideas about Indian culture and health practices. In the eyes of many Anglo-Americans, Indians suffered from disease, not from a lack of immunities or from external circumstances, but because of inherent weaknesses attributable to their place in the evolutionary scale of human progress. Anglo-Americans not only viewed Native Americans as morally, culturally, and socially backward, but also regarded them as weak in body. In a way, the myth of the disappearing Indian acted as a self-fulfilling prophecy that allowed white Americans and the United States government to ignore disease and death on reservations since whites deemed the act of disappearance as the inevitable fate of all native people.

The self-fulfilling nature of the disappearance myth led Anglo-Americans to believe that they could silence native voices on many different levels. Confinement to reservations placed Indians under constant surveillance and persistent pressure to assimilate into the dominant society. Anglo-Americans—whether missionaries, bureaucrats, academics, or others—often talked of "killing the Indian" and creating a "white" person out of Indians. Death was the ultimate means of fulfilling the mission of wiping out the presence of native cultures in the United States. But death not only worked to destroy culture; it also physically silenced those voices seeking to maintain the integrity of Native American culture and life. Anglo-Americans allied themselves with death on the reservations. They may have been saddened by the loss of life, but the larger project of assimilating Indians and consuming their culture was served by Indian deaths.

Anglo-Americans viewed the death of Indians as part of the inevitable demise of Indian cultures. They also used death as a means to obscure the unpleasant and violent nature of conquering many different peoples. If those whom you conquered no longer exist to remind you of the bloody and violent acts that you committed, then it is much easier to create and maintain a mythos that glorifies your past. Indians played a crucial role in this mythos. They were the antagonists, the impediment to be surmounted and conquered on the way to fulfilling Manifest Destiny. Native peoples made the story heroic and allowed Anglo-Americans to view the conquest of Indian lands as an act filled with courage and valiant deeds. When their role was finished, Indians were to disappear from the stage, either through death or assimilation. In reality, Anglo-Americans confined Indians to reservations not for their protection, as many bureaucrats and reformers stated, but as a way to silence them, either through physical death or assimilation. It did not pay to have physical reminders of the brutality of one's actions. Living Native Americans haunted non-Native Americans, particularly through historical studies, so it was better to erase their presence from the earth. Although Americans have been reluctant to admit it, the United States government and white settlers committed genocide against Yakama people and their neighbors, and the statistical evidence provided here confirms the results of the genocide during the tragic years of the reservation era.

White Americans not only wished to physically silence native people through their assimilation or death, but they also silenced them by framing death in a substantially different way. For most whites, whether Protestant or Catholic, death meant the end of physical life, as well as the promise of judgment and retribution for a person's deeds on earth. The death of a non-Christian Indian meant the ultimate silencing of pagans or heathens, since Christians believed that unbelievers were sent to hell and suffered eternal punishment for their sins. This view often clashed with native peoples struggling to maintain their own ideas of death and the afterlife. Each side viewed death and its consequences differently, leaving little room for Anglo-Americans to comprehend Indian practices and beliefs. Failing to understand or appreciate the complexity and depth of Native American views of death and its importance also led Anglo-Americans to misunderstand that for Native Americans the way one died often created very important implications for how death was handled and what ceremonies needed to be performed for the deceased, their family, and the community as a whole. This lack of understanding translated into a disregard for any of the physical manifestations associated with the death of a native person. Anglo-Americans ignored and silenced practices regarding death just as they silenced all other parts of Indian culture and life. For whites, Indian death and the ways that native people understood it was incomprehensible and unimaginable, except in the simplified way of relegating non-Christian Indians to the realms of "heathen" unbelief and damnation.

Disregard for native beliefs also took on a physical dimension as government officials, white doctors, and medical institutions intervened in the lives and health care of native peoples on reservations. Living on a reservation brought all Indian life, ritual, and practice, including activities surrounding the death of individuals, under the surveillance of whites on the reservation. Anglo-Americans often frowned on traditional death practices and sometimes forced these practices into the periphery or underground. The issue was further complicated as some Indian people on the Yakama Reservation converted to Christianity and struggled with competing views of death. Christian Indians faced pressure from Indian agents, missionaries, and their fellow Christians to abandon all practices associated with the nontraditional community, including ceremonies performed for the dead for thousands of years.

Forgotten Voices is an effort to rectify this silencing of an element of Native American history as it relates to the Yakama Reservation in Washington State. Despite the best efforts of bureaucrats, doctors, reformers, politicians, and non-Indian populations, the Yakama who lived in the late 19th and early 20th centuries can still tell us how they lived and died if we listen carefully. In order to understand what they are trying to tell us, it is important to know the history of the Yakama people. How the Yakama lived their lives shaped the way that they dealt with death. In order to help the reader understand how Yakama people gave significance to and responded to death, a brief overview of their lives on the Columbia Plateau follows.

The "Yakama"

Many tribes compose the contemporary Confederated Tribes of the Yakama Nation. Historically, the people spoke several dialects of three separate language families, including Sahaptin, Salish, and Chinook. Yet the people of the Columbia Plateau shared many cultural elements. For the purposes of this study, we will focus on the Yakama, the largest group living on the reservation today, although we understand that citizens of the Yakama Nation have the blood of many different peoples flowing through their veins.

The Yakama people and their neighbors have lived, worked, traveled, and died on the Columbia Plateau for thousands of years. The Yakama homeland stretched over large portions of the Columbia Plateau. The western boundary reached into the Cascade Mountains. Mount Adams and Mount Rainier, both part of a chain of dormant volcanoes, were sacred places for Yakama people, both spiritually and economically. The Yakama hunted game and gathered roots and plants in the Cascade Mountains. To the east, Yakama territory extended well into the Columbia Plateau, reaching and overlapping into the Walla Walla, Snake, and Palouse River valleys. The southern boundary of Yakama territory was formed by the Columbia River, where the Yakama maintained extensive fishing sites. Most Yakama and their neighbors lived in semipermanent villages and towns located along streams and rivers in the region, in particular the Yakima Valley. The Yakama people were divided into two principal groups, the Lower and Upper Yakama. The Lower Yakama lived east of the Cascades in the lower portion of the Yakima Valley. They formed the largest portion of the population. The Upper Yakama, sometimes called the Kittitas, occupied the upper valley, living in seven villages. During a large part of the year, the Yakama moved from place to place hunting, gathering, and fishing for food sources like camas, khouse, berries, moss, salmon, deer, elk, and a number of other plants and animals found on the Columbia Plateau.[1]

The Columbia Plateau is a unique geographical region, principally known for its aridity and undulating hills cut by the Columbia River. Many newcomers considered the Columbia Plateau a desert unsuitable for human habitation, but native peoples, including the Yakama, had survived and thrived in the region for thousands of years. A native son of the plateau, Donald Meinig, authored of one of the most influential studies on the Columbia Plateau.[2] He noted that the landscape and climate of the region shaped the human geography of the area. The lack of large game animals, like the buffalo, and the minimal small game and plant life made subsistence on the plateau difficult. The one source of consistent food lay in the rivers of the region like the Columbia and Snake rivers. Annually these rivers carried millions of salmon to their spawning grounds and provided native peoples in the region with one of their most important sources of food. Additionally, Native Americans point out the rich plant life of the region that provided them with roots and berries, sometimes in great abundance. For the Yakama and their neighbors, the salmon, deer, roots, and berries were sacred, and the people celebrated the holy gift through First Foods Ceremonies, which they continue to offer in the tradition of the Washat. The patterns of life on the plateau created a situation where native peoples like the Yakama used the region in a seasonal pattern. Wintering on the fringes of the plateau, where there was less snow and the temperatures were warmer, the Yakama prepared for the seasonal round that occurred during the spring, summer, and fall months.

The seasonal round, as practiced by the Yakama and other Columbia Plateau communities, formed the basis for survival and activity throughout the year. Each season required strenuous effort, planning, and organization in order for communities to survive during the winter. The arrival of spring was generally marked by people traveling to annual root grounds to gather nutritious bulbs. They left the root grounds when they learned that the first Chinook salmon run had begun. Yakama people moved from their villages to fishing sites located mainly along the Columbia River, harvested the fish, and then moved on to other sites where women harvested roots and berries for eating and storage. Among the favorites were camas, bitterroot, khouse, wild carrot, and wild onion. The concentration of these roots in specific locations led to the interaction of many different Indian communities. Yakama, Nez Perce, Umatillas, and other communities met to gather roots, hunt, and interact on a social, political, and cultural basis. In this way, young people met their future spouses and formed permanent familial relations. Horse racing, gambling, games, storytelling, arranging of weddings, and many other activities also occurred during these times. The Yakama and their neighbors sang and danced together, forming economic, familial, and spiritual bonds that remain intact today.[3]

By late June and early July, the rivers in the region dropped sufficiently to expose summer runs of salmon, and Yakama people, along with many other native groups in the region, returned to fishing sites to harvest salmon. When the salmon runs slowed, women switched their subsistence activities to gathering more plants and berries, while men hunted deer, rabbits, birds, and other small animals. In the late summer months, starting in mid-August, families moved to camps located in the high country surrounding the Columbia Plateau to harvest the very rich black mountain huckleberry fields, often remaining there until the beginning of October, "the time when the tamarack turned yellow."[4] As the late fall approached, the Yakama returned to their winter villages and prepared for this season by laying in as much food stores as possible, including last-minute hunting and fishing.[5]

During the winter months, Yakama people prepared for the arrival of spring by repairing tools and equipment. There was also plenty of time for storytelling, the education of young people, visiting relatives, and planning for the next seasonal round. One of the most important activities of the winter months was the winter dance or Guardian Spirit Dance. The winter dances provided an opportunity for young people in the community to exhibit and demonstrate their newly formed relationship with a guardian spirit and also allowed the community to discern the power and gifts given to individuals through this relationship.[6]

The winter dance or Guardian Spirit Dance was a religious ceremony that held great significance for the Yakama and other Indian communities on the Columbia Plateau. The dance was the culmination of a long process of education, storytelling, and questing that brought young people into contact with spiritual beings. These spiritual beings formed relationships with a young person that lasted throughout their lives and the relationships also imbued the youth with certain powers and abilities crucial for the survival of their community. Families and communities carefully prepared their children for this encounter with the spirit world since approaching a guardian spirit without proper preparation could result in disease, accident, or even death. Preparation for the quest often included sweat baths, prayer, fasting, and exercise. After proper preparation, adults took young people to secluded sites in a location with spiritual significance for their family or community. During this seclusion, a "guardian spirit" established a relationship with the young person, teaching him or her songs, dances, and proper etiquette to maintain the relationship. For example, Kamaikin, one of the best-known Yakama leaders, sought his *tah*, or guardian spirit, on the slopes of Mount Rainier. During his seclusion, a buffalo visited Kamaikin and shared its power with him. Once the young person established this relationship with a spiritual being, he rarely discussed the experience in public. Spirit seekers generally visited shamans or medicine people to help them understand the nature of their power and to discuss any difficulties or improper manifestations of their power. Young people usually sought their *tah* power in the fall of the year at the end of the seasonal round.[7]

Movement of the people to and from sacred places, root grounds, and hunting areas changed with the domestication of the horse during the 18th century. The horse allowed the Yakama and other Indian communities to expand the seasonal round and also transport more food and material over greater distances. Not only could Yakama people conduct the seasonal round with more efficiency, but they also expanded hunting expeditions across the Bitterroot Mountains to find buffalo, often hunting with their relatives and friends the Nez Perce, Palouse, and Spokanes. The ability to hunt buffalo also brought the Yakama into greater contact with Indian communities east of the Bitterroot Mountains, including potential enemies. Yakama hunting parties came into greater contact with Salish-speaking Flathead people, as well as Shoshone, Blackfeet, Paiute, and other Mountain and Plains tribes.

While the Columbia Plateau was not the most hospitable area in the Pacific Northwest, the region offered some protection from outsiders, both Indian and European. The Yakama and other Plateau communities maintained an almost continual state of warfare with Shoshonean peoples to the south, often called the "Snake Indians" by white settlers. These Shoshonean-speaking groups often raided the plateau and stole horses from Plateau groups. However, the Shoshone received horses in the mid-18th century, before the Plateau people received them, giving the Shoshone an advantage militarily. Living in the Inland Northwest also afforded some protection from diseases introduced by Europeans at the end of the 18th century, but with the horse came a smallpox epidemic from the Great Plains. Disease also entered the plateau from the Pacific Coast, traveling up the Columbia River and its tributaries. Contact with Plains and Coastal Indian communities led to the introduction of smallpox, malaria, influenza, and other communicable diseases in the Columbia Plateau. Yakama people suffered greatly from these initial epidemics, losing nearly half their population. Even though the Yakama met Euro-Americans later than other Indian populations in North America, they still felt the impact of Euro-American presence through epidemics, horses, and firearms, often before directly meeting the newcomers.[8]

Yakama people heard about and met Europeans before the arrival of the Lewis and Clark expedition of 1805. Their proximity to and trade with Coastal Indian communities led to the meeting of Euro-Americans before other Plateau communities. Even with this previous experience, the arrival of the expedition marked a new era for the Yakama and their neighbors on the Columbia Plateau. For the first time, the Yakama interacted and negotiated with representatives of the United States government. Yakama leaders met with the Lewis and Clark expedition along the Columbia River before the expedition arrived at The Dalles. For their part, the Yakama were interested in learning about Anglo-Americans as potential allies and trading partners, as well as being motivated by curiosity. Both parties remembered the meeting fondly, and the Yakama hoped that the good relations established by the Lewis and Clark expedition would continue in their further contacts with the United States and its citizens.

Unfortunately, the initial good feelings did not continue. In the 1830s and 1840s, missionaries arrived from the United States, bringing Christianity to the Yakama and other Plateau communities. Marcus and Narcissa Whitman, Henry and Eliza Spalding, and a number of other newcomers traveled to the Oregon Country in response to reports of a delegation of Nez Perce that traveled to St. Louis to find out about the white man's book of power, the Bible. The Board of Foreign Missions recruited missionaries for the Oregon Country and dispatched them with the goal of converting Native Americans on the Columbia Plateau. Protestant and Catholic missionaries came to the Yakama and sought to convert them to Christianity. Initially, the missionaries enjoyed the hospitality and good feelings of the Plateau Indian communities, but this situation did not last long. Missionaries Marcus Whitman, Henry Spalding, and others managed to anger the people they worked with, either through acts of arrogance like the imposition of Christian and American laws on native communities, or by encouraging white settlement and migration through the territories of Plateau Indian communities. Non-Indian immigration also brought disease, including a devastating measles epidemic in 1847. Anger was expressed in 1847 when members of the Cayuse tribe killed Whitman, his family, and many others at the mission. After the murders and the ensuing military action, Protestant missionaries such as Spalding left the Northwest and would not return to Yakama land until later in the 19th century. However, Catholic missionaries continued to preach among the Yakama during the 19th century.[9]

As white settlers continued to stream into the Oregon Country, the U.S. government decided that the so-called Indian Question needed addressing. In 1854, Congress appointed Isaac I. Stevens as territorial governor and superintendent of Indian Affairs for the newly formed Washington Territory, with the express purpose of extinguishing Indian land claims to large parts of the territory. Stevens directed numerous treaty councils with many different native communities throughout the Pacific Northwest, but the treaty negotiations with the Yakama and other Columbia Plateau Indian communities occurred in the Walla Walla Valley from May 29 to June 16, 1855. During the treaty deliberations, Stevens and Oregon's superintendent of Indian Affairs, Joel Palmer, antagonized and belittled many of the Indians present, but despite these slights, representatives from most of the Plateau communities agreed to sign three treaties, including the Yakama Treaty. Great dispute still surrounds the role of Kamaikin at the Walla Walla Council. Stevens insisted that Kamaikin signed the treaty, therefore extending the provisions to the Yakama and Palouse. Kamaikin, on the other hand, placed his mark on the treaty as a sign of peace and friendship, but he never would have claimed to represent all the Yakama, Palouse, or other Indians party to the Yakama Treaty of 1855. The treaty created three reservations. The Yakama Reservation was not exclusively set aside for them but also included people from other Indian communities like the Wishram, Palouse, and others. Through the treaty, Plateau Indian communities ceded nearly sixty thousand square miles of territory to the U.S. government. The resentment and anger created by the Yakama Treaty, coupled with Anglo-American violations of the treaty provisions, quickly led to violence and warfare between the U.S. government, the Yakama, and a number of other Plateau Indian communities.

Between the fall of 1855 and the spring of 1858, the so-called Yakama War raged across the Columbia Plateau. With the discovery of gold north of the Spokane River, Indian lands on the Columbia Plateau faced continual trespass by miners attempting to reach and exploit the gold fields. Miners stole horses, murdered Indians, raped women, and violated the provisions of the Yakama Treaty, a treaty not ratified until 1859. The U.S. government failed to address these violations, and when two Yakama men murdered Yakama Indian Agent Andrew Jackson Bolon, the United States sent troops into Yakama territory to quell what whites believed to be Indian aggression in the Oregon Country.

Fighting continued off and on from the fall of 1855 to 1858. The Yakama were only one of many Indian communities involved in the fighting. Many Palouse, Cayuse, Walla Walla, Umatilla, Coeur d'Alene, and Spokane communities also took part in the fighting. Kamaikin played an instrumental role during the last part of the war, often acting as unifier since he was related to important Palouse, Nez Perce, and Spokane families. Two major campaigns by the combined forces of the United States Army and territorial volunteers from 1855 to 1857 failed to defeat Indian resistance on the Columbia Plateau. The third and final campaign, commanded by Colonel George H. Wright, started in the summer of 1858. While Wright never decisively defeated Indian forces, the pressure of his campaign divided Indian communities into two groups, one desiring peace negotiations and the other wishing to continue the struggle. In the end, the battles of the Four Lakes and Spokane

Plains demoralized the Yakama, Palouse, and their allies, leading to greater confusion and dissension. After the battles, Wright and his men marched through the eastern part of the Columbia Plateau, accepting the surrender of numerous Indian communities and imposing the will of the U.S. government on the Columbia Plateau. Colonel Wright and his men also executed a number of Indian leaders, including Owhi and Qualchin, important Yakama headmen. As a result of the war, the U.S. Army occupied large portions of the Columbia Plateau and created new forts and military installations to monitor and control the Indian peoples of the region.[10]

Ratification of the Yakama Treaty and the end of the so-called Yakama War in 1858 opened most of the Pacific Northwest to white settlement. After the war in 1859, Congress ratified the treaty concluded at the Walla Walla Council. In that same year, the Office of Indian Affairs (or Indian Office) developed the structures and policy for the reservation reserved for the Yakama and 14 other Indian tribes, including the Palouse, Wishram, Wenatchee, and others. According to the provisions of the 1855 treaty, the United States guaranteed the borders and land of the reservations and agreed to protect native peoples from white aggression and trespass. The Office of Indian Affairs controlled nearly every aspect of life on the reservation. Indian people confined to the reservation struggled with conditions that they found there. Whites continued to trespass on reservation land, steal Indians' livestock, and exploit tribal water and timber resources. Settlers often refused to allow the Yakama access to important root, berry, hunting, and fishing areas, thus destroying the native economy, which was closely tied to the physical, social, and spiritual well-being of the people.

Yakama people on the reservation faced many challenges as Anglo-Americans forced programs of assimilation onto the people. Some Indians converted to Christianity, while others followed the Washani, Feather, or Indian Shaker faiths. Whichever faith one adhered to, Yakama people continually dealt with federal agents, missionaries, and white reformers attempting to "civilize" or assimilate them into Anglo-American society. One of the most visible aspects of this assimilation campaign was the establishment of a school at Fort Simcoe in 1859, designed to teach young boys and girls how to fit into American society. Parents, grandparents, and other relatives who resisted the attendance of their children at the school faced fines and imprisonment. The assimilation program also included efforts to force the Yakama to take up farming since this was deemed a civilized occupation and a way to erode traditional Indian subsistence patterns. While some farming occurred, the Yakama and many other Inland Northwest Indian peoples continued to follow older patterns of life, but with ever greater difficulty because white settlers and businesses increasingly owned the land where these activities had previously taken place.

While the Yakama struggled to adjust to reservation life, the U.S. Congress passed the Severalty Act in 1887 as a further attempt to assimilate Indians across the continent into Anglo-American society. Under the so-called Dawes Act, government agents usually allotted 160 acres of land to each head of family and smaller portions of land to single people, orphans, and other categories of Indian people. The U.S. government held this land in trust for twenty-five years. At the end of this time, the allottee received a fee patent and owned the land free and clear, which meant that Indians had to pay taxes on their land. The government, white reformers, and churches believed that twenty-five years was ample time for Indians like the Yakama to learn to farm their land and that ownership of land would accelerate their assimilation into Anglo-American society.[11]

In 1892, Special Allotting Agent John K. Rankin arrived on the Yakama Reservation and began the process of assigning allotments. Rankin made 1,817 allotments, finishing his work in June 1894. The Yakama retained around 440,000 acres in individual allotments and 780,000 acres in commonly held tribal land. The allotment process was only one of many steps in the long course of taking land from Yakama people. Starting with the Yakama Treaty of 1855, the Yakama and all other Plateau communities relinquished huge tracts of land. After allotment, Yakama people continued to lose their land through sale, debt payment, and swindle by white Americans. Today, white Americans own over half of the allotted acres of the former Yakama estate. Not only did the Yakama lose their land, but they also did not become farmers as hoped by white reformers and the U.S. government. The process of land loss was accelerated as the U.S. government opened the reservation to white settlement after allotment. Struggling with the loss of land and inundated by white settlers, the Yakama fought to maintain their identity and property throughout the early 20th century. They also dealt with consequences of confinement to the reservation, including poverty, poor health, alcoholism, and diseases like tuberculosis, diabetes, influenza, and pneumonia. Like many other Indian communities prior to World War II, the Yakama death rate, both adult and infant, rose dramatically compared to the larger general population of the United States.[12]

While issues of land retention and loss consumed both Indians and Anglo-Americans, other property, like fishing sites and rights, emerged in the 20th century as crucial areas to test the limits of treaty rights and to encourage self-determination. Yakama people, like many other Columbia Plateau communities, maintained fishing sites along the Columbia River, principally at The Dalles and Celilo Falls areas, but also along many smaller streams in the region. Indian people occupied these sites for thousands of years, and the treaty reaffirmed the right of Indian peoples to take fish "at all usual and accustomed fishing places."[13] As the United States confined more and more Indian people on reservations, white settlers, farmers, ranchers, and fishermen occupied many of the areas along the Columbia River and other important salmon fishing streams. Along with occupation of fishing sites, whites introduced fishing techniques like the fish wheel that dramatically increased the size of salmon harvests and therefore affected the ability of native people to use their fishing sites effectively. As whites took more fish and moved onto traditional fishing sites, conflict exploded between the two groups. Matters became worse when state game and fish officials arrested Indians for fishing without state licenses and out of season. Early in the 20th century three federal court cases upheld tribal fishing rights along the Columbia River and its tributaries. Each of the cases involved Indians from the Yakama Nation who were pushed off of their traditional fishing sites by fish wheel operators. While the courts consistently ruled in favor of Indian fishing rights, their rulings failed to clarify the issue of state regulation of Indian fishing off the reservation. Both Washington State and Oregon passed legislation to limit the amount of salmon taken and they outlawed certain forms of fishing on the rivers.

Faced with competition from whites and interference from state governments, Yakama people continued to fish, as best they could, from their traditional sites. From 1938 to 1968, the U.S. Army Corps of Engineers built a series of dams on the mid-Columbia River. These dams significantly impacted salmon runs and traditional fishing sites. In 1957, the federal government flooded the fishing areas of the Celilo Falls on the Columbia River. Yakama people, along with many other Pacific Northwest Indian communities, struggled to maintain their fisheries and traditional methods of procuring salmon. Due to the construction of dams and competition from white fishermen, most Indians along the Columbia River saw their catches decline. In the midst of this crisis, tribes attempted to find a solution that allowed for an equitable distribution of catches. After much litigation, the Yakama and many other Indian communities in the Inland Pacific Northwest won a significant court case in 1969 known as the Boldt decision that guaranteed tribes a 50 percent portion of harvestable salmon.

The struggle to maintain land and fishing rights coincided with ever stronger efforts to exercise sovereignty and self-determination on the reservation. While the Office of Indian Affairs controlled almost all aspects of life on the reservation, Yakama people contested this control and eventually exercised greater control over their lives and property. One of the turning points in this struggle came during the Great Depression with the passage of the Indian Reorganization Act of 1934. The Yakama declined reorganization, but they formed their own government in 1935. Each of 14 different tribes on the Yakama Reservation elected a representative to the tribal council. At the age of 18, all enrolled Yakamas become members of the General Council. At present, there are approximately 8,800 enrolled members of the Confederated Tribes and Bands of the Yakama Nation.

On a daily basis, members of the Yakama General Council and the tribe as a whole do not focus their attention on infectious diseases and the deaths that stalked tribal members in the past. The Yakama people have new and important business to address, including the current health issues of their tribal members. However, much has changed since the early 20th century, when infectious diseases plagued the tribal people and caused so many deaths. Elder Yakama people know about this time period and the devastating diseases that took the lives of so many of their people. The elders remember the deaths of many loved ones, infants, and children who passed away from bacterial and viral maladies that are generally under control today. Scholars have been remiss in studying disease and death during the reservation period of American history and exposing the continued deaths that visited Indian people after the Indian and American wars, forced removals, and confinement on reservations. This study offers original data that expose the depth of disease and death on one reservation at the very time the government of the United States attempted to assimilate Indians and destroy Native American cultures. *Forgotten Voices* is a product of over twenty years of work in assembling the data and analyzing them. Some of the more compelling data are provided in this book for use by future scholars who wish to use the statistics and compare them with new data sets from other reservations.

Forgotten Voices is a data set drawn from Yakama death records found in the National Archives, Pacific Northwest Branch, in Seattle, Washington. The records include a few death registers kept by agents working for the Office of Indian Affairs and, more importantly, death certificates authorized by the state and created by Yakima County health officials with the help of Indians and non-Indians from the Yakama Reservation. The documents included 3,899 cases, available for the years 1888 to 1964. During the 22-year period from 1888 to 1910, federal employees and Yakima county officials recorded 29 deaths of people from the Yakama Reservation, which is a gross undercounting of the number of deaths on the reservation. Washington became a death registry state in 1907, but Yakima County officials did not make a concerted effort to record Indian deaths on the Yakama Indian Reservation until 1924. Before the 1920s, Yakama Indian agents made little effort to collect copies of death documents from state officials responsible for recording deaths on the reservation, and they made little effort to fulfill their duties to keep vital statistics on births and deaths as mandated by the federal government in 1884. The Office of Indian Affairs did not make a concerted effort to record deaths among Yakama people until the 1920s, when the Brookings Institute began a large investigation into the Indian Office. Although incomplete for the early years, data included in this volume for the 76-year period are a rich source of information, providing a unique opportunity to study mortality over time on one Indian reservation. Scholars have published little on the reservation era of the Yakama and other Plateau Indians, and less on deaths over time on the Yakama Reservation. Yakama death certificates provided a way in which to study a poorly documented element of American Indian history. The statistics found here will enlighten researchers and provide them data from which to draw their own conclusions.

Over the years, Yakama people have not been studied historically in terms of mortality. In part this is because of the absence of a data set from which to study the fourteen different tribes and bands that once lived on the Yakama Reservation.[14] These Indians included Yakama, Klickitat, Wenatchi, Wanapum, Wasco, Wishram, Palouse, and others, but death certificates identified nearly all Indians living on the reservation—regardless of their tribal backgrounds—as "Yakama." Researchers cannot identify one tribe from another within the data set or compare statistics related to each tribal group. Since no similar data set exists from death certificates or death registers focusing on another reservation, no comparative study can be offered. However, perhaps the publication of this data set will encourage other scholars to initiate comparable studies and offer their data sets. Scholars may compare some of the data with the general population of Washington State, whites in the United States, African Americans in the United States, and nonwhites in the United States. However, a better understanding of Native American mortality will occur after other scholars create data sets of deaths over time on other reservations and compare their findings with this Yakama data.

The data found in this volume suggest that Yakama mortality history is related to the theoretical framework created by Abdel R. Omran, a professor of medicine at the University of North Carolina. Omran's work on epidemiologic transition suggests that the Yakama data fit into four overlapping transitional periods: (1) Pre-Euro-American Contact, (2) Age of Pestilence and Famine (ca. 1800–1920s), (3) Age of Receding Pandemics (ca. 1900–1940s), and (4) Age of Degenerative Man-Made Diseases (1940–present).[15] The first period is beyond the scope of this study, but the second period began before the arrival of Meriwether Lewis and William Clark in 1805, when European disease became more pronounced among Northwestern Indians.[16] The Age of Pestilence and Famine proved disastrous for the Yakama and their neighbors, as smallpox, malaria, measles, diphtheria, fevers, and other contagious diseases ravaged native populations. During this era, a variety of viruses and bacillus invaded Indian peoples, killing indiscriminately. On the reservations and beyond, tuberculosis, pneumonia, and influenza also spread among Native Americans, killing large numbers of people. This was particularly true toward the end of the 19th century. By 1900, many of these diseases retreated among some American populations, but tuberculosis, pneumonia, and influenza grew in importance as causes of death among the Yakama. During the Age of Receding Pandemics after 1900, smallpox, malaria, and measles withdrew as important causes of death, but tuberculosis, pneumonia, and influenza caused many deaths. Tuberculosis became the primary killer.

Yakama death certificates provide insights into these causes of death as the Age of Pestilence merged with the Age of Receding Pandemics during the first decades of the 20th century. Tuberculosis became the most important cause of death on the reservation from 1924 to 1944, when the disease declined rapidly in importance. Bacteria cause tuberculosis, but human hosts become more susceptible when their bodies lack nutritious foods. Furthermore, environmental and educational factors on the Yakama Reservation also contributed to a tubercular epidemic during the early 20th century. The Yakama Reservation lacked an education system to teach the emerging field of public health and sanitation. In addition, Indian populations forced to the reservation lacked quality housing and sewage systems. Poverty plagued the Yakama Reservation, and the Office of Indian Affairs failed to provide the Yakama with medical doctors and nurses trained to isolate and treat tubercular patients. The Indian Office also failed to establish a sanitarium on the reservation. All of these factors contributed to the rise in deaths caused by tuberculosis.

Deaths caused by tuberculosis declined in the 1940s, in part because of health officials who identified and isolated TB patients. In addition, citizens of the Yakama Nation understood the disease and permitted their loved ones to be sent to sanitariums, usually the sanitarium at Fort Lapwai, to recover from the illness and to be isolated from the healthy. In the 1940s, the Yakama entered a new era when tuberculosis, gastrointestinal disorders, and pneumonia declined in importance as central causes of death. After World War II, the Yakama entered the Age of Degenerative Man-Made Diseases when heart disease, cancer, and accidents became the primary causes of death on the Yakama Reservation. Although it is beyond the scope of this study and the data presented here, records from the Indian Health Service on the Yakama Reservation indicate that during the late 20th century (1980s and 1990s), alcohol-related deaths, diabetes, accidents, pneumonia, murders, and suicides became important causes of death among Yakama people. Thomas McKeown, Barry Popkins, and other scholars have argued that part of this transition to man-made disease is a predictable product of nutrition related to "modernization." The data seem to indicate that this is the case among Indians living on the Yakama Reservation. Indeed, Yakama people lost nearly all their daily required traditional foods by the 1940s, and after World War II, consumed refined foods that they purchased with cash earned through labor, leases, and family businesses.[17]

The data found here are particularly strong regarding the cause and number of deaths on the Yakama Reservation. It is revealing in terms of infant and childhood mortality. Two prominent scholars, Samuel Preston and Michael Haines, have maintained that "the single most valuable piece of information for predicting child mortality is the mother's race."[18] Since Native Americans constituted all of the cases recorded in the death certificates on the reservation, this data will be of value to demographic historians in general, as well as those interested in Native American history.

Some scholars have argued that once the United States forced Indians onto reservations, a large number of Indians—but most markedly infants and children—died as a result of the reservation system. Unfortunately, data on population, disease, infant mortality, and death rates do not exist for the period prior to the reservation system, so no comparison can be made regarding Yakama deaths prior to 1855, when the United States established the reservation through the Yakama Treaty. Prior to white contact, as noted by Lewis and Clark, Yakama people suffered eye ailments and they died from several causes, but few people died from communicable disease, except from occasional epidemics. Although the Indians of the Columbia Plateau did not live a utopian life prior to white contact, their standard of living was relatively high most of the years due to healthy diet, climate, housing, and resources. Most of the tribes, even those speaking diverse language families, coexisted in peace, sharing food resources, geographical areas, spiritual beliefs, and ceremonies. The people generally spoke other Indian languages and intermarried with each other, forming familial relationships that exist to this day. According to John R. Weeks, director of the International Population Center and noted scholar, "prior to European contact mortality rates were high, but more predictable." He argues that people "knew what to expect as causes of death, even if they identified them differently than does the Western medical model. Predictability is, of course, a staple of human existence."[19] However, contact with Euro-Americans

> brought unknown diseases—a strong element of unpredictability—and even though immunity to these diseases would likely be developing within one or two generations, the cultural traditions have no basis for identifying these causes of death and so they remain culturally unpredictable, which may help account for the anomie and other symptoms of distress—beyond those that would naturally be associated with being penned into a reservation.[20]

By using the Coale-Demeny model life tables, some suggestions can be made regarding pre-European-American-contact death rates. Weeks argues that "if we assume that the average Yakama was producing 5 live births (a little less than average for pre-modern women throughout the world), and that the population was growing slowly (0.5 percent per year—positive, but not widely perceptible in the short-term), then the life expectancy would had to have been about 30 years for women and about 28 for males." Under these conditions, females would have had a crude death rate around 38 per 1,000 in the Yakama population and males about 33 per 1,000. "The general fertility rates (babies per 1,000 women of reproductive ages) would be about 84." Furthermore, Weeks points out that if the above assumptions were correct then "the implied infant mortality rate is about 300 per 1,000 live births, and about 40 percent of all deaths will be children under the age of 5." Weeks concludes by stating that if fertility were higher or growth slower, then death rates would have been higher. But if the growth rate was slower prior to contact, there would be a lower death rate.[21]

Contact with Euro-Americans brought on the Age of Pestilence that devastated native populations in the Northwest. The spread of disease and continuance of unhealthy conditions were made worse by government policies designed to confine large numbers of diverse tribes and bands onto single land areas where the Office of Indian Affairs could control and convert them to white "civilization." A common hypothesis presented by historians argues that government Indian policies forced Native Americans from their traditional lands and ruined economies. This occurred during the Age of Pestilence and Famine when the government of the United States concentrated a number of Indians onto limited acres of tribal lands, designating these areas as reservations. The government sought to change Indian economies, making native peoples "civilized" through agriculture. Agents expected Indian people to eke out a living as farmers (and later ranchers) on a small portion of their former estates, and in competition with other tribes and bands placed on the same reservation. These developments harmed native communities in many ways, particularly the health of people through the destruction of diet and nutrition.[22]

During the late 19th and early 20th centuries, Native Americans had to compete for their livelihood with non-Indians who resettled former Indian lands. These newcomers often changed the environment by ranching, farming, mining, irrigating, fencing, and road-building. Newcomers destroyed natural resources such as game, fish, roots, berries, and timber, and the results proved disastrous for Indians in terms of diet and religion, since they had a spiritual relationship to plants, animals, and places. Many times government agents prevented Indians from hunting, fishing, and gathering off the reservation, in spite of treaty rights, because originally agents wanted all Indians to become farmers tied to the soil. During the Walla Walla Council, Governor

Isaac I. Stevens made it clear that Indians could continue to hunt, fish, graze, and gather on and off the reservation, but by the early 20th century, agents of the federal, state, and county governments in the Northwest tried to prevent native people from exercising their natural and treaty rights. In the mid-20th century, employees of the Office of Indian Affairs joined forces with state officials with the force of law, and tried to prevent Yakama and other Indians from exercising their rights to hunt, fish, and gather at all usual and accustomed areas on and off the reservation.[23]

Under the terms of the Yakama Treaty of 1855, Indians secured for themselves their age-old right to fish, hunt, and gather. Stevens said as much in the Council minutes, and according to the Yakama Treaty, Indians could fish at all usual and accustomed areas, which included sites outside the reservation boundary.[24] All this was understood by Indians and whites at the time of the Walla Walla Council. Prior to the establishment of the reservation, Yakama men, women, and children followed a seasonal round, fishing and gathering roots in the spring and summer, hunting in the fall and winter, and gathering berries in the summer and fall. Yakama and other Plateau Indians had practiced very limited farming prior to the reservations, since the earth held a bounty of natural foods that did not require cultivation. Agriculture on the Columbia Plateau had never been a major component of native economies. The demand by the Office of Indian Affairs that the Yakama should become farmers was difficult at best and actually contrary to their spiritual beliefs that required them to eat specific foods at certain times of the year to celebrate and give thanks for these foods in holy feasts. In sum, the general policy of the Office of Indian Affairs was to force Yakama Indian people to remain on the reservation and make their livelihood through agriculture rather than by traditional means. Other agencies of the federal government aided in this effort by placing dams on Northwestern rivers and restricting the movement of Native Americans to hunting, fishing, and root grounds. Without the opportunity to hunt, fish, and gather as they had in previous years, the health of the Yakama Indians suffered and people died as a result.[25]

Housing became another factor that affected the health of Indians on the Yakama Reservation. On most reservations, Indians had to live in nontraditional housing because of limited resources. Indians, like the Yakama, who were accustomed to traveling about in seasonal rounds, setting up and bringing down their homes continuously, were forced to remain in the same geographical area for large periods of time. This was a dangerous development and impaired the general health of Yakama people. Traditionally, Yakama people lived in mat lodges, mat-covered tipis, and buffalo hide tipis. When they resided in their permanent village sites, they used their large A-framed mat lodges. When the seasonal round began in the spring, they dismantled these lodges and moved to early root grounds, using their tipis for housing. This system of seasonal rounds fostered hygiene, since the Yakama set up and dismantled their homes many times throughout the year and moved from place to place. Each time they moved, they cleaned their dwellings and policed their village sites. During the late 19th century, the people no longer moved across the plateau changing their homes. Instead, they lived in settled hovels that became breeding grounds for viruses and bacillus, particularly tuberculosis, that spread rapidly within the homes. Tubercle bacillus spread from sputum that traveled through airborne dust and partides to infect humans. The bacteria generally entered the respiratory system of its host, but it could also land on eating utensils, blankets, pillows, clothing, pipes, and other material items and enter the body through the nose or mouth. Upon the death on an individual, Yakama custom required the people to give away all of one's belongings, including material items infected with bacillus. The disease spread and tuberculosis became the foremost killer of the Yakama from 1924 to 1944.[26]

As a result of the reservation system, the Office of Indian Affairs encouraged Indians to remain on the reservation for most of the year. Resettlement of the Columbia Plateau by whites, the building of dams, the settlement of non-Indian tubercular patients in Washington, and the destruction of the natural foods familiar to the Yakama mitigated a change in lifestyle and housing. Whites farmed, ranched, and logged many regions of the Columbia Plateau, changing the environment, which was detrimental to Indians. Rather than moving about for a good portion of the year, the Yakama became confined to the reservation, where they lived in mat lodges and small wood-framed dwellings throughout the year. With time, some of these dwellings became overcrowded and unsanitary, most of them having dirt floors. The health of Yakama people suffered from inadequate sanitation, absence of clean ground water, rivers polluted by insecticides, and complete lack of any means for treating sewage. The change of housing among the Yakama contributed to their ill health, and the people became ill and died.[27]

When Indians became ill, the Indian agency on the Yakama Reservation was poorly prepared to take care of them. No hospital existed on the reservation until 1928, and the government never established a sanatorium for native people of central Washington or Oregon. Nearly all Yakama tubercular patients relocated to the sanatorium on the Nez Perce Reservation. Agents lacked adequate medicines, medical staff, and hospitals to care for the people. The Yakama Reservation encompassed over one million acres, and the lack of transportation on the part of Indians and medical staff prevented people from traveling to Toppenish, White Swan, or Fort Simcoe to receive medical care. Traditional knowledge of curing procedures and medicinal plants was kept by elderly men and women, not herbal specialists. They were educated in the ways of the Yakama and commonly treated people before and after the establishment of the reservation. Traditional treatments continued to be used to fight eye problems, infections, wounds, and pain. However, Yakama people faced new biological enemies that did not respond to old treatments. Elders employed their knowledge but found these methods ineffective in controlling tuberculosis, pneumonia, heart disease, measles, influenza, and syphilis.

Medicine men and women, trained to deal with different forms of "spirit sickness," were also unable to control these new diseases. It was a hopeless situation for the people on the reservation, and Yakama society fell into a general anomie, as the people were usually unable to heal themselves, control the new diseases, or cope with the grim reality resulting from the numerous illnesses and deaths suffered by friends and relatives on the reservation. Stress caused by rapid cultural, economic, political, and social changes cannot be quantified, but the large number of deaths on the reservation suggests that stress was a major factor in the ill health of Yakama people. The role of medicine men and women diminished over the years, in part the result of the general breakdown in traditional culture resulting from the reservation system, forced assimilation, and government policies. Before the arrival of whites, medicine men and women—especially midwives or birthing doctors knowledgeable about pregnancies, nutrition, birth, delivery, and postpartum care—healed people and provided preventive and curative information. These people had less influence after the arrival of "white man's diseases" that did not always subside when treated with traditional medicine.

Before the invasion of the Northwest by whites, Yakama people became ill from spirit sickness, contact with powerful totems, violations of sacred places or procedures, and witchcraft. They also died from a number of physical causes, including infections, accidents, war, heart failure, cancer, etc. However, the white invasion brought the Age of Pestilence, with new diseases, environmental change, cultural dislocation, and sociopolitical upheaval, all of which contributed to the deterioration of health conditions. According to Abdel R. Omran, epidemiologic transactions contributed to "the destruction of group cohesion, the rise of mental illness, crime, delinquency, drug dependency [including alcohol]," and cultural anomie. In addition, he argued that populations were weakened by stress, hypertension, and suicidal tendencies.[28] As one person stated, "We get sickness from white man: measles, chickenpox, smallpox, whooping cough, flu, and all from white man."[29] Thus, the arrival of newcomers significantly changed the causes and cures of disease introduced by non-Indians. In addition, the reservation system and inadequacies of the Office of Indian Affairs generally contributed to the poor health of Native Americans on the Yakama Reservation. An analysis of the statistical data taken from the death certificates recorded for the various Indians on the Yakama Reservation makes this clear.

Unfortunately, no body of data regarding deaths on the Yakama Reservation is available for the years from 1859, when the United States created the Yakama Reservation, to 1888, when the agents collected the first death records for the Yakama Reservation. The Yakama censuses of the 1880s note a few deaths, simply by indicating "dead" beside a few names. However, it is unclear what year the person died, since the censuses run from July 1 to June 30 and they do not state the primary and secondary causes of death. Because of the lack of accurate and detailed data, no accurate comparisons can be drawn with the early 19th century, when the Yakama suffered from epidemics of smallpox, measles, and influenza. The death data between 1888 and 1911 are poor, and the data kept by the Office of Indian Affairs between 1912 and 1923, although better, are not complete. However, the data kept after 1924, when Indians became citizens of the United States and when Yakama agents responded to national Indian reforms, dramatically increased. The present study is an examination of the available death data, principally death certificates preserved by the Office of Indian Affairs after 1924, in order to analyze the cause and number of deaths on the Yakama Reservation, including infants and small children. Admittedly, this is a narrow examination of one reservation, primarily using a single data source of 3,889 cases. However, the database assembled for this study is unique. It is the first ever assembled from death certificates on the Yakama Reservation, and it deals with a lengthy period of time. Although the data from 1888 to 1924 are weak, it represents a portion of the 3,899 cases kept at the National Archives for Yakama people and for this reason it is used in this study.

The work offers an aspect of Yakama history never before examined, and it may encourage other scholars to employ similar sources and methods in analyzing the history of native peoples. The intent was to focus on reservation people, not urban Indians or those who filed Indian homesteads off the reservation, although many of the families who once owned homesteads or lived in urban areas joined their friends and relatives on the Yakama Reservation during the course of the 19th and 20th centuries. Most of the Indians who filed homesteads were Wenatchee, Palouse, Wishram, and others, but not Yakama, since most Yakama secured for themselves a portion of their former homelands. No attempt was made to identify and discover death certificates for members of these families, who had homesteaded along the Columbia and Snake rivers, for to do so would be a monumental task. These people were largely full-bloods—often peoples of mixed Native American heritage—and not usually Indians of mixed Indian and white blood. No one should assume that because an Indian family filed a homestead that they were not full-bloods or that they considered themselves any less "Indian" because they filed a "legal" claim to their traditional homes. This was not the case. However, this study on death provides an in-depth work on one reservation over a period of 76 years, focusing on the social history of numerous Indian people living on a single reservation.[30]

Although the agency letterbooks, tribal censuses, and reports to the commissioner of Indian Affairs sometimes mention deaths, death registers and certificates offer the best information on mortality. Agents at the Yakama Agency made no concerted effort to collect and preserve death registers until 1888. The present study is based on the 3,899 death certificates preserved in the National Archives, Pacific Northwest Region, in Seattle, and the documents range over a period of time from 1888 to 1964. The earliest death data collected by county and state officials from 1888 to 1923 are poor and suggest the lack of attention paid to their required duty of collecting vital statistics. However, the data collected after 1924 are excellent, offering insights into the number and causes of death as well as other variables, including gender of the deceased, place of death, tribal affiliation, and blood quantum. The Yakama Agency kept death registers and certificates that indicate that the Yakama experienced one death per year for the period from 1888 to 1905 and from 1907 to 1909. Yakama Agency officials preserved records indicating three deaths in 1906 and six deaths in 1910. By any measure, these are low numbers, and they do not reflect the actual and, unfortunately, unknown number of deaths during the late 19th century and the early 20th century.[31]

Agents on the Yakama Reservation began collecting more information after 1910. This may have been the result of the Progressive Era in the United States and a renewed interest in the welfare of Native Americans, particularly by Commissioner of Indians Affairs Robert G. Valentine.[32] The trend to gather better data and record them might also have been linked to the General Allotment Act as agents applied allotment to the Yakama Reservation in the early 20th century. Under the terms of allotment, the United States divided a portion of the Yakama Reservation into individual allotments of 160-, 80-, and 40-acre parcels, depending on the age and marital status of individuals. In order to allot the reservation, agents required an accounting of all Indians living on or near the reservation, and agents conducted censuses on the Yakama Reservation. Censuses also served as the basis for funding a particular reservation, so the more people that agents listed on the censuses as Yakama living on the reservation, the more funding the agency received. Death certificates provided the Office of Indian Affairs with another means of tracking Indians who were no longer within the Yakama population and who would not be allotted.

As a result of the Progressive Era and the General Allotment Act, the Office of Indian Affairs developed an interest in collecting better data on the Yakama Reservation, and record keeping with regard to the death certificates on the reservation improved. However, the best vital statistics on the Yakama Reservation came later in the 20th century in response to another more profound reform movement. Even so, the data appears to be incomplete, particularly with regard to deaths for children under one year of age during the years between 1910 and early 1920s. Simply put, parents did not report the deaths of their babies to white agents or Indians working at the agencies. Families simply buried these babies, keeping the burials quiet, familial affairs. Although inadequate, the death certificates after 1910 indicate a new interest on the part of the Office of Indian Affairs to collect copies of death certificates, thus recording a larger number of deaths. The death certificates after 1920 provide the most complete information of the deceased person's name, age, sex, and cause of death.[33]

Overall, the Office of Indian Affairs acquired the most number of death certificates on the Yakama Reservation between 1924 and 1941, an era that corresponded with a major national reform movement in American Indian affairs.[34] This reform era is briefly presented below.[35] The reforms began, in part, as a result of a grant from John D. Rockefeller, Jr., to the Institute of Government Research—renamed the Brookings Institute. In 1926, the Institute launched a major investigation into the condition of Native Americans in terms of their health, education, and economy. In 1926, Lewis Meriam began his research that culminated in 1928 with the publication of *The Problem of Indian Administration*, commonly called the Meriam Report. The book was a revealing work that fueled the fires of national reformers. It examined many aspects of Indian life, including health, and provided a good deal of valuable information on Indian health and mortality.[36]

According to the Meriam Report, "taken as a whole practically every activity undertaken by the national government for the promotion of the health of the Indians is below a reasonable standard of efficiency."[37] Meriam also commented on the failure of the Office of Indian Affairs to meet minimum standards of governmental health care. "The health work of the Indian Service," Meriam wrote, "fall[s] markedly below the standards maintained by the Public Health Service, the Veterans' Bureau, and the Army and the Navy, and those prescribed to the states by the national government in the administration of the . . . Maternity and Infancy Act." Furthermore, Meriam noted that a major problem in analyzing the health of Indians in the United States was the poor records collected and kept by the Indian Office. He reported that "for many years" the agencies "had rules and regulations requiring the collection and tabulation of vital statistics." However, after an exhaustive search through the records of several Indian agencies—including the Yakama Agency—Meriam found that "accurate figures based on reasonably complete records are not yet secured."[38]

In his landmark report, Meriam wrote that "many of the Indian deaths which occur on reservations" went unrecorded since "no report is made to the Indian Office." Furthermore, he maintained that when agents had collected death certificates, the information on the documents was "defective in that some of the essential items are missing." Meriam had studied death certificates "with a view to learning the relative importance of various conditions in producing deaths" but he soon found that in large numbers of the death certificates "a statement of the cause of death was missing."[39] This is in reference to 11 reservations surveyed for their death records, none of which was the Yakama Reservation. However, the statement is accurate with regard to the Yakama Reservation. Meriam further argued that since it was "a generally accepted axiom today that the quality of a service is accurately reflected in the completeness and accuracy of its records," that it was factual to say that "the Indian Service has been weak."[40]

Meriam maintained correctly that "the statistics and records of medical activities at present are incomplete and unreliable."[41] Unfortunately, this is all too apparent in the records kept by the Yakama Indian Agency. The death records for the Yakama Reservation are incomplete, but they represent the only major data available on the subject and are valuable sources of information on the causes and numbers of death on one Indian reservation. Meriam's study began in the early 1920s when white reformers of Native American affairs in the United States demanded that the government investigate conditions on the reservations. The research committee led by Lewis Meriam was a direct result of their demands. The government published the Meriam Report in 1928, the year before the stock market crash and the onset of the Great Depression. Reform of American Indian affairs stalled until the election of Franklin D. Roosevelt, who selected John Collier as his commissioner of Indian Affairs. Collier kept this post until 1946, pressing forward with numerous national reforms in Indian affairs, including health, education, tribal government, and economic development.[42] This was part of the Indian New Deal. Statistics kept at the Yakama Agency show a dramatic improvement in the number of deaths recorded and the completeness of the documents from 1924 to 1964, and this is a result of the national reforms, not an increased number of deaths on the reservation.

The agents, doctors, and other employees working at the Yakama Agency performed an inadequate job of collecting documents or reporting deaths to county and state health officials so that death certificates could be made. However, the information is descriptive and clinical, not medical. No record has been found to suggest that doctors performed autopsies, so we have no medical descriptions of death. Dr. H. De Lien and J. Nixon Hadley pointed out that "twenty years ago, it was a common practice to allow the reservation superintendent, who was not medically trained, to inscribe on the death certificate his surmise as to the cause of death."[43] In 1952, these authors argued that the agency "doctor is frequently requested to assign a cause for a case that occurred 200 miles away and for which he has only hearsay evidence, sometimes supplemented by a previous hospital record." As a result, doctors frequently recorded the death, stating that the cause was unknown.[44] Although death certificates collected with the help of agency physicians were flawed in relationship to cause of death, the data provided by these documents "represents the best available information of the person best-trained to make the determination, but is subject to an unknown percentage of error."[45]

Federal and state officials were derelict in their duties to collect accurate and complete death certificates for several reasons. For one, white officials working for the state and federal governments were dealing with Indians, people who some non-Indians considered backward, uncivilized, barbaric, and unprogressive. To some, Indians were the "vanishing race," and some whites viewed Indian deaths as a natural consequence of interfacing with an "advanced civilization." Some agents, including well-meaning Christians, viewed the death of Native Americans under their care as an embarrassment to themselves, the Indian Office, and the nation. If the nonnative public of the United States knew the actual number of Indian deaths, they might have demanded greater and more far-reaching reforms than they did in the early 20th century. Americans may have demanded new leadership in Indian affairs, forcing agents and superintendents from their entrenched positions.

On the Yakama Reservation, none of the agents serving from 1888 to 1910 considered the collection of vital statistics regarding Indian deaths to be a priority, or if they did, they did not convey their conviction to those responsible for collecting data. Agents and their employees managed all of the business associated with the reservation, and they did not focus their attentions on recording vital statistics. Perhaps they were preoccupied with issues involving agriculture, irrigation, fishing, education, road building, timber harvests, land allotments, law enforcement, trade, and others. Agents certainly busied themselves "civilizing" and Christianizing Indians. They were a part of a huge bureaucracy that dealt in paper—writing letters, taking censuses, completing forms, and filing reports. They likely did not champion the task of tracking Indian deaths, especially on a land base as rural and as large as the Yakama Reservation with a population roughly ranging from two thousand to three thousand people.[46] Furthermore, some employees of the Indian Affairs Office felt that the duty of dealing with vital statistics was one that involved counties and states, not federal agencies. Transportation and communication systems were not well developed on the reservation, making it difficult for county, state, and federal officials to learn about deaths that occurred some distance from agency headquarters at Fort Simcoe or Toppenish. Between 1888 and 1910, officials of the Indian Office made little effort to record deaths of the "vanishing race" in any area of the reservation, including that region surrounding Fort Simcoe.[47]

In addition to governmental inefficiency, Indians themselves lacked information regarding deaths within their own communities. Sometimes long distances separated Yakama people from the agency. Poor transportation and communication systems worked against any effort on their part to report deaths. However, many Yakama people resented the government of the United States for its control of nearly every aspect of tribal affairs. Most likely few Yakama wished to cooperate with white bureaucrats by sharing their most personal grief with agents who had dictated policy to them since 1855. This was particularly true regarding parents who lost fetuses and infants, since families and friends quietly mourned these deaths in their own fashion, burying the children without notifying agents. When deaths occurred, one of the last things on the minds of Yakama families was to notify the county, state, or agency officials so that white bureaucrats could record an Indian death.

As a result of many factors, death certificates do not represent the full range of deaths that occurred on the Yakama Reservation from 1888 to 1964. Federal and state officials sometimes learned of the death of elders since their funerals brought large numbers of Indians to a particular area to mourn. Usually the death of an important man or woman resulted in an outpouring of gifts and participation by larger Northwestern Indian communities. The death of a fetus, infant, or child, however, did not attract as many people, particularly those from other reservations, and some of these deaths and burials went unnoticed and unrecorded by the state. Still, a large portion of the known deaths were those of children, which leaves one only to imagine the actual number of fetuses, infants, and childhood deaths that the government never recorded.

Death certificates and registers for the Yakama Indian Reservation are not complete, but they represent the best information available regarding deaths among Yakama people from 1888 to 1964. Some individual family members kept oral and written accounts of deaths in their families, but copies of the Washington State death certificates kept for the Yakama Agency are the most complete recorded information available regarding deaths on the reservation during this 76-year period. This study is based on these documents, with individual descendents as the unit of analysis. This work is an attempt at a census, rather than a sample, of Yakama deaths, since it considers the death of every person that officials recorded through death certificates or registers. The statistics found in this volume include cause of death, year of death, age at death, gender, and place of death. We also provide the explanation of death as found on the death certificate. Clearly, the data presented here tell us something of mortality on the Yakama Indian Reservation, offering some of the voices of those men, women, and children who died on the reservation from 1888 to 1964.

Variables

The data presented in this volume are derived from death certificates for the Yakama Indian Agency on file at the National Archives, Pacific Northwest Region, Seattle, Washington. The authors have provided all the copies of death certificates used in this study to the Yakama Tribal Library, Toppenish, Washington, and researchers may find copies of all the death certificates in both locations, as well as the originals on file with Washington state officials.[48] We have carefully considered which variables to use, and we have selected cause of death, year of death, age, gender, and place of death. These are the variables found in this data set. We present the cause of death in the data set as explanation, since this is the variable designation given on the documents, and we chose to replicate the wording found on each death certificate. As a result, researchers will be able to view the exact wording of the cause of death or explanation in this data set, including the different ways officials described the various causes of death for Yakama people. These are clinical explanations of death, not medical explanations, since the Yakama Agency, to our knowledge, authorized no autopsies or lab tests. This is an important factor, particularly with regard to tuberculosis and pneumonia. It is highly likely that since tuberculosis was so prevalent among the Yakama that many of the infant and childhood deaths reported as pneumonia were likely tuberculosis, which could infect an infant or child and destroy the body very rapidly. Of course, we have no way of knowing this today, but it is likely that tuberculosis and not pneumonia killed far more infants and children than reported.

The cause of death or explanation is the means of organization, and the causes are the central focus of the data set. We feel that the most important variable found in this work was the cause, and we provide some analysis of some of the major causes of death in the introductory narrative, including tuberculosis, pneumonia, heart disease, gastrointestinal disorders, influenza, cancer, premature births, and old age. We also included the data from several other causes of death, including kidney disease, hemorrhage, childbirth (deaths of mothers, infants, and fetuses indicate an infant death), whooping cough, stillborn, venereal disease, blood poisoning, exposure, surgical complications, bronchitis, paralysis, liver disorders, typhoid, measles, suffocation, encephalitis, and appendicitis. However, in this data set, we omitted four causes of death, including miscellaneous accidents, automobile accidents, murders, and suicide, all of which are dealt with in Clifford Trafzer's *Death Stalks the Yakama*. The authors are continuing to refine the research and statistics on these causes of death and will create a separate study of them in the future. We will present a discussion of each variable below and begin with cause of death.

Cause of Death

The most important variable in this study was cause of death, and it was a nominal variable. We developed numeric codes for each discrete cause of death, and we coded cases accordingly. In cases where death certificates listed more than one cause of death, we assigned the case the numeric code corresponding to the first or primary cause of death listed on the death certificate. Since the study begins in 1888, no attempt was made to analyze deaths prior to this date. Unfortunately, since data for deaths during the Age of Pestilence of the 19th century is not available for the Yakama, we provide no serious comparisons between the causes of death in the 19th and 20th centuries. It is known from the historical literature that smallpox from trading vessels arrived in the Northwest in 1775, and it came up the Missouri River and Great Plains, spreading death in 1782 to 1783, 1801, 1824 to 1825. This disease killed a large but unknown number of Indians in the Northwest, as did "fever and ague." The "Cold Sickness," or influenza, also killed a number of Indians in epidemics, and in 1847 a measles epidemic ravaged the Cayuse and other Indians of the Inland Northwest.[49] No data are provided regarding these causes of death among Yakama people prior to 1888, since they are not within the scope of the study.

Omran has pointed out that "scattered accounts of epidemics leave no doubt of its existence in the eighteenth and parts of the nineteenth century." These epidemics included "intermittent fever (now malaria), typhoid, influenza, measles, parotitis, scarlantina, smallpox, syphilis, thrush, whooping cough, and yellow fever. Consumption (tuberculosis), pneumonia, and bronchitis were grouped under respiratory diseases."[50] Epidemics of some of these spread among Plateau Indians, but no accurate records exist regarding the numbers of people who died of these scourges. Moreover, during the era of this study, tuberculosis, influenza, pneumonia, bronchitis, and whooping cough killed Yakama people in large numbers. Yet information taken from death certificates indicated that these are only five of the eighty-seven causes of death coded from the Yakama data base, and this study only provided data for the more important causes of death. By 1888, smallpox and measles were insignificant killers of Yakama people, but other causes of death—particularly tuberculosis and pneumonia—plagued the people, bringing death throughout the early 20th century.

Several causes of death occurred only a few times in the data set, including "arthritis," "bad cold," "diphtheria," "epilepsy," "fever," "gonorrhea," "rickets," and "carbuncle." Minor causes of death will not be addressed in the work. Unfortunately, of the 3,899 cases reported in the data set, the cause of death of 1,082 individuals (28 percent) is unknown, unrecorded, or illegible in the death certificates. Several of the death certificates simply did not include the cause of death or included the statement "Not Known."

Several other death certificates had a handwritten cause of death, but the writing was not legible. If the statement was illegible, the authors coded the person's death as unknown. However, we made every effort to read these difficult causes of death with a magnifying glass and consult with colleagues. The large number of unknown, unrecorded, and illegible statements regarding the cause of death represents poor or careless record keeping on the part of county and state officials or agents and reservation doctors who were required by state law to keep vital statistics and aid in the collection and preservation of accurate statistics.

In coding the cause of death, we recorded one cause of death for every individual. In some cases, county and state officials recorded the primary and secondary cause of death on the death certificates. In such cases, we coded only the primary cause of death, but made note of secondary causes of death in our data set. For example, if the person died of pneumonia but also had tuberculosis, which probably contributed to the onset of pneumonia, we coded for pneumonia, not tuberculosis. Likewise, if a person died in an automobile accident but was intoxicated, we coded the person's death as an automobile accident but noted that the accident was alcohol-related.[51] We recorded the secondary causes of death in our data set, but make no attempt to analyze the secondary causes. In order of presentation, the major causes of death include tuberculosis, pneumonia, heart disease, gastrointestinal disorders, influenza, cancer, premature births, and senility and old age.

Tuberculosis

The most frequently recorded cause of death among the Yakama from 1888 to 1964 was tuberculosis (n = 619, or 28 percent), and it preyed on the Yakama until its decline in the 1940s. Usually the disease develops slowly and is caused by airborne bacilli that spread from one person to the next. It was prevalent on the Yakama Reservation because of abject poverty suffered by this native population. Confinement on the reservation and dwindling natural food resources off the reservation left Indians with less to eat. Processed foods did not provide the bodies of Yakama people with the same nutrients as traditional foods. Furthermore, confinement to the reservation led to banishment from former root, hunting, and fishing areas. Life on the reservation led Indians to live in permanent homes that were less sanitary than temporary mat lodges and tipis that the people continually built and rebuilt throughout the year. The reservation system encouraged poverty, ill health, and death. The Office of Indian Affairs did little to address these ills. The reservation offered a breeding ground for bacilli and viruses that caused tuberculosis, pneumonia, gastrointestinal disorders, and other maladies. The Yakama between the ages of 15 and 29 suffered the most deaths resulting from tuberculosis on the reservation. Cows also carried tubercle bacteria, and the disease was transmitted through milk often given to Native American children at school. However, Yakama people did not drink large quantities of cow's milk because most were allergic to cow's milk. Tuberculosis usually traveled through the air to infect Yakama people. It was characterized by a dry cough accompanied by phlegm, pus, and blood. Victims generally suffered fever, fatigue, and loss of appetite. Persons affected by the disease often lost weight and developed lumps in their body. Tuberculosis could attack various parts of the body, including bones, brain, and kidneys. Most often it spread to the lungs, where the bacilli multiplied, inflaming and destroying the tissue of the affected area.

Tuberculosis acted in two stages, the first being a bacterial attack on a particular part of the body that then counterattacked through its defenses. For several months the body's antibodies surrounded and attacked the bacteria, but generally some of the tubercular bacillus escaped and moved through the blood to other areas. Antibodies corralled the bacteria in the new area, and this process could repeat itself for months. Antibodies simply contained the tubercular bacteria, but they did not necessarily kill them. For this reason, the tubercle bacilli could become active at any point. This was particularly true if the person became undernourished, weak, depressed, or ill from another disease, which was a common condition on the reservation. Thus, in the death records for the Yakama, county and state officials sometimes recorded that people had secondary causes of death, in addition to the tuberculosis. Secondary causes of death included heart disease, syphilis, influenza, and meningitis. Undoubtedly, these contributed to tubercular deaths on the Yakama Reservation.

The second phase of tuberculosis was often referred to in the death certificates as "consumption." The body's defenses were not sufficient to contain bacilli, and they began to grow at an alarming rate, taking over an organ or parts of the body. If the lungs became infected, the person had trouble breathing. If tuberculosis spread to other parts of the body, the disease could become active there as well, particularly if the person was weakened by poor diet or secondary infections.[52]

Tuberculosis was the principal killer of Yakama Indians between 1888 and 1964, and it was an important disease in the United States into the 1950s. Tuberculosis was listed as the cause of death for 619 (28 percent) of the Yakama people. It likely killed many others whose cause of death was listed as "unknown." Furthermore, tuberculosis probably killed most of the children and infants that officials recorded as pneumonia deaths, because tuberculosis could be very aggressive in children, particularly infants, whose weak bodies could not fight the bacterial infection. Since the agency did not conduct autopsies, we have no way of knowing the medical cause of deaths, but medical specialists of upper respiratory diseases suggest that since tuberculosis was the prevalent disease among the Yakama, most likely infants and children died of tuberculosis, which authorities mistakenly recorded as pneumonia. The disease ravaged the Yakama population until the 1940s, when a dramatic change occurred. Health officials on the Yakama Reservation controlled tuberculosis through isolation of patients and education so that during the period from 1950 to 1964, it killed only 13 Yakama people.

Sometimes deaths by tuberculosis were complicated by pneumonia or a malady identified by physicians as pneumonitis. However, in most cases, the officials recording adult Yakama deaths through the death certificates provided specific descriptions of the disease, including "pulmonary tuberculosis," "tuberculosis of bones," and "glandular tuberculosis." Sometimes people with tuberculosis suffered complications brought on by other diseases, including "tuberculosis and pneumonia," "tuberculosis and meningitis," and "tuberculosis and syphilis." Tuberculosis was a devastating disease, and it was the leading cause of death on the Yakama Reservation.[53]

Pneumonia

Like tuberculosis, pneumonia flourished on the Yakama Reservation because of poor housing, inadequate diets, lack of sanitary knowledge, and insufficient medicine and medical staff (n = 566, or 26 percent). Pneumonia was usually caused by viral or bacterial infections, but it could also result from chemicals like poison gas. However, unless a Yakama individual was exposed to gas in World War I, it is unlikely that this was a factor causing pneumonia on the Yakama Reservation. Pneumonia brought on by influenza or tuberculosis was dangerous. For Indians lacking natural immunities and suffering from malnutrition, depression, or other diseases, viral pneumonia was extremely deadly.

In general, two major types of pneumonia exist: lobar pneumonia and bronchopneumonia. Lobar pneumonia is characterized by an inflammation of one lobe of one lung that could spread to other lobes. In bronchopneumonia, the inflammation began in the bronchioles and bronchi—airways—and spread to tissues in one or both lungs. The most common form of bacterial pneumonia was streptococcus pneumonia, although other forms of bacterial pneumonia included hemophilus influenzae, legionella pneumonphilia, staphylococcus aureus, and others.[54] Pneumonia was commonly characterized by inflammation of the lungs, but it included many other inflammations. Part or all of one lung might be affected or both lungs could contract pneumonia. Individuals with the disease often coughed, exhibited high fevers, suffered chills, sweated profusely, and complained of chest pains. They could be short of breath while resting, and they could cough phlegm that contained blood. Sometimes children with pneumonia had a blue tint to their skin and lips. People with the disease sometimes suffered delirium, and in severe cases, they died. This was particularly true of patients with tuberculosis, heart disease, cancer, and bronchitis. This could also be the case with someone who had had a stroke. Thus, officials at the Yakama Agency often diagnosed pneumonia as the immediate cause of death, when the person was previously stricken by some other illness.[55] In addition, officials likely ascribed pneumonia as the primary cause of death, especially of infants and children, when in fact they died of tuberculosis, which can strike and kill children relatively quickly when the bacterial disease is so prevalent within a population.

Many death certificates indicate that the person simply died of pneumonia, but in some cases, the documents describe the deaths as "pneumonia and influenza," "pulmonary pneumonia," "pneumonia following measles," and "lobar pneumonia." Of the 3,899 people reported to have died between 1888 and 1964, a total of 566 (26 percent) reportedly died of pneumonia. Pneumonia was a foremost cause of death. Pneumonia arrived with Euro-Americans. Indeed, even though immunity to these diseases would likely be developed within one or two generations, the cultural traditions have no basis for identifying these causes of death and so they remain culturally unpredictable, which may help account for the anomie and other symptoms of distress—beyond those that would naturally be associated with being penned into a reservation.

Living on the reservation changed the ability of Yakama people to fight off diseases like pneumonia. Depression and anomie accompanied people through their everyday lives, compromising their immune systems and making it harder to fight off infections. Increased infection rates of tuberculosis, influenza, and other communicable diseases set the stage for greater pneumonia risk. Often Yakama people recovered from one infection only to be stricken with pneumonia because their immune system was weakened. With the advent of antibiotics in the 1920s and 1930s, medical practitioners for the first time effectively treated patients with bacterial pneumonias. As antibiotic use increased, deaths from pneumonia dropped in the general population. On reservations, the death records tell another story. Yakama people continued to die from pneumonia during the 1950s and 1960s—22 percent of pneumonia deaths recorded in this study occurred during these decades. While health services improved for Indian people on reservations after World War II, it is clear that the effects of decades of poor treatment, poverty, and insufficient medical care would have a lasting legacy among the Yakama people.

Contact with Euro-Americans brought on the Age of Pestilence that devastated native populations in the Northwest. Pneumonia raged among Yakama infants and children under six years of age. Many more Yakama male infants died of pneumonia than females, but this is common among infants in general. According to Charles B. Clayton, writing for the American Medical Association in the *Encyclopedia of Medicine*, pneumonia "is more common in males, during infancy and old age." However, Clayton does not explain why.[57] José Jorge Clor de Alva, former professor of ethnic studies at University of California, Berkeley, has suggested that more Yakama male infants than female infants died of pneumonia because of child abuse. There is no cultural, historical, or social evidence to support such an assertion.[58] During the 1940s and 1950s, pneumonia continued to cause deaths on the Yakama Reservation at the very time that government health services controlled tuberculosis. During the 14-year period from 1950 through 1964, pneumonia caused the death of 125 Yakama people. A total of 22 percent of all deaths caused by pneumonia occurred during the last 14 years of this study.[59]

Heart Diseases

Heart diseases of all kind, including heart disorders, diseases of the valves, heart attacks, heart failure, congenital heart disease, and others, represented the third leading cause of death among the Yakama during the late 19th and early 20th centuries (n = 325, or 15 percent). Tobacco use was not an extremely common practice among Yakama before World War II, and therefore smoking did not contribute greatly to heart disease prior to the 1950s. Instead, heart disease was linked to diet, which changed dramatically during the course of the 20th century from native fruits and vegetables to processed foods, including government commodities. According to Barry Popkin, director of the University of North Carolina, Chapel Hill, Interdisciplinary Obesity Center and the Nutrition Epidemiology Division, changes in diet are related to "modernization" and they shift patterns of mortality. One such dramatic change among Yakama people included the rise in heart disease after World War II which, in part, resulted from changing diets and the loss of nutritionally valuable foods after the war.[60] Nutritional and dietary changes also affected pregnant mothers and their children. "Many females," according to Omran, "developed pelvic deformities with rickets which led to later difficulties in childbirth and higher rates of maternal death."[61] Poor diets weakened the health of many people, including pregnant mothers, who sometimes gave birth to children with heart diseases. Heart attack was a major cause of death and was characterized by blockage caused by blood clots in coronary arteries that cut off the supply of blood to one region of the heart muscle and damaged that part of the heart. Generally the clot was caught in the blood vessel, because the artery had atheroma or fatty deposits within the artery that narrowed and restricted the flow of blood. Someone suffering from a heart attack often has severe angina in the chest, neck, jaw, arms, and stomach. They may also experience shortness of breath, chills, fainting, nausea, sweating, and dizziness. A heart attack could be fatal if it impeded the electrical impulses that regulate the heart or if damage to the heart was severe.[62]

Heart failure affected Yakama Indians, and weakened heart muscle or valves impaired the pumping of the heart, making the organ inefficient. When this happened, heart failure occurred. When the heart could not pump normally, blood collected in the vessels and flowed either into the lungs or other parts of the body, overloading these areas with excess blood. Heart failure stressed the entire body, and it was fatal. When a Yakama woman was pregnant, her heart worked harder than normal. If the mother had a heart disorder, including a murmur, the difficulty of the prenatal period or childbirth could be fatal.[63]

Babies also suffered from congenital heart disorders or abnormalities of the heart at the time of birth. Congenital heart disease could result if the mother had an infection, particularly German measles or rubella. A fetus could develop heart problems during the first three months after conception, and the cause could not be known. Between 1888 and 1964, government officials recording Yakama deaths reported that only 2 percent of all children who died between birth and age five died of heart disease. However, heart disease was the third largest killer of all Indians on the Yakama Reservation during the 76-year period, causing the death of 325 people (15 percent). During the 1940s and 1950s, while tuberculosis declined rapidly as a major cause of death among Yakama people, heart disease became the leading killer on the reservation. Between 1950 and 1964, heart disease claimed the lives of 127 people. Of all Yakama who died of heart disease during the last 14 years of this study, 29 percent died as a result of heart disease. Washington state officials recorded the deaths of Yakama from heart disease in many ways, including "heart failure," "arteriosclerosis," "organic heart disease," "pulmonary edema," and "pulmonary hemorrhage." In addition, officials sometimes reported secondary causes of death associated with heart disease, including "heart disease and premature childbirth," "heart and renal disease," and "heart disease and pleurisy." Heart disease was a significant cause of death on the Yakama Reservation, particularly after 1950, when it became the leading cause of death.[64]

Gastrointestinal Disorders

The fifth major cause of death in the general Yakama population was gastrointestinal disorders (n = 124, or 6 percent). Problems of the stomach, intestines, and other organs of the digestive tract proved fatal to adults and children alike, particularly if infections developed. Prior to 1930, antibiotics were not available on the reservation, and medical staff on the reservation often found themselves short on antibiotics during the years after the 1930s. Although the digestive tract naturally contained necessary and vital bacteria, harmful bacteria sometimes invaded the body where they multiplied rapidly, infecting the gut wall and entering the bloodstream. Dangerous bacteria can spread to other areas of the body, including other parts of the digestive system, and they proved harmful and deadly to a person.

Nearly all infections of the digestive tract were caused by bacteria, and infants could ingest bacteria from unsterilized bottles, clothes, and unclean parts of another's body, particularly unclean breasts and unwashed hands. Infants are particularly vulnerable to bacilli contracted from fecal material. People infected with gastrointestinal disorders presented one or more symptoms. They often exhibited general intestinal and abdominal pains, cramps, vomiting, fever, and diarrhea. Usually, a person suffering from gastrointestinal disorders became thirsty, but they often had difficulty keeping fluids in their stomachs because of vomiting. The malady was complicated by diarrhea that contributed significantly to the person's state of dehydration.[65] Disorders of the stomach, intestines, and other parts of the digestive tract accounted for 124 deaths (6 percent) in the general population. Officials recorded deaths resulting from gastrointestinal disorders in many different ways, including "stomach trouble," "bowel trouble," "intestinal obstruction," "entero colitis," "astroenteritis," "choleliathiasis," and "accute [*sic*] enteritis."[66]

Influenza

Influenza became the seventh leading cause of death on the Yakama Reservation—a disease often identified as flu (n = 104, or 5 percent). Many varieties of influenza viruses existed and they were continually evolving, with new strains developing all the time. Influenza was an airborne disease that generally spread when an infected person coughed or sneezed. The virus entered the body of Yakama people through the upper respiratory system—the nose and mouth—and it most often traveled into the lungs. Within days after contact, a person might show symptoms such as sneezing, coughing, sore throat, chills, chest pains, head and muscular aches, and high fever.[67] Medical doctors and state recording officials sometimes linked influenza and pneumonia, but most often they recorded "influenza" as the primary and only cause of death, describing influenza in death certificates as "Spanish influenza," "intestinal influenza," "influenza since birth," and "grippe." At times, recording officials linked influenza to other causes of death, and some death certificates stated that Yakama people died of "Spanish influenza and tuberculosis," "influenza and pneumonia," "flu and senility," and "influenza and choletithitis."[68]

Epidemics of influenza occurred on the Yakama Reservation, spreading to many Indians and killing some. Historically, influenza was a major killer of Native Americans in general and Northwestern Indians in particular. It was sometimes labeled the "Cold Sickness" by white observers, and it devastated entire villages along the lower Columbia River. In 1827 and 1829, Northwestern Indians suffered from a strain of influenza from Asia. The disease caused a horrible epidemic that traveled from the coast of present-day Washington and Oregon into the interior. The flu moved up the Columbia River and its tributaries, killing Indians indiscriminately. The "Cold Sickness" took its toll among many tribes, including Indians living on the banks of the Columbia and Yakima rivers. The Yakama were not spared. In 1918 the Yakama suffered the effects of the Spanish influenza, a strain of the influenza virus that infected and killed people throughout the United States. Interestingly, the Spanish influenza killed few infants and children, but rather preyed on the elders of the Yakama Nation. Between 1888 and 1964, influenza caused the death of 104 Yakama people of all ages (5 percent).[69]

Cancer

The eighth leading cause of death on the Yakama Reservation was cancer, including all varieties of the disease. According to the death certificates, Yakama people died of many types of cancer affecting the stomach, liver, lungs, cervix, uterus, breasts, bladder, blood, intestines, rectum, pancreas, and other parts of the body. Specifically, the death certificates reveal several types of cancer that took the lives of Yakama people, including "uterine cancer," "carcinoma of cervix," and "carcinoma of liver."[70] Cancer is a disease usually characterized by cells multiplying and spreading uncontrollably. Cancer can develop in any part of the body and result in a malignant tumor. Cancer can spread from one area to the next, affecting vital organs. It can develop in blood, muscle, liver, lung, bladder, brain, or other parts of the body. It is not always deadly, but cancer treatment during much of the era under discussion was not well developed.

On the Yakama Reservation, cancer contributed to the deaths of far more women than men (n = 58, or 71 percent), and women died most often of uterine, cervical, stomach, and breast cancer.[71] These forms of reproductive cancer were major killers of Yakama women between 1888 and 1964, but neither men nor women suffered severely from lung cancer. Indeed, lung cancer claimed the lives of two females and three males during the 76 years of the study, and the reason is likely the lack of tobacco use among the Yakama prior to World War II. The people considered tobacco a sacred plant and used tobacco ceremonially. Most people did not smoke tobacco on a daily basis. During the 76 years of the study, only five Yakama died of lung cancer, but cancer of all kinds killed 82 (3 percent) Yakama Indians. Significantly, although cancer was a leading cause of death on the Yakama Reservation, it was not as important a cause of death as it was among whites, nonwhites, or the people of Washington State during the same period.[72]

Premature Births

Premature birth was the ninth leading cause of death on the reservation, and it only killed fetuses (n = 64, or 3 percent). Prematurity was described as the birth of a baby before 37 weeks' gestation. This cause of death contributed to the loss of a large number of infants on the Yakama Reservation, particularly the deaths of male babies, who suffered more from premature births than did females. Males also died in larger numbers than females from stillbirths. Stillbirths and premature births led the causes of death for Yakama fetuses. The death of these children resulted in large part from the ill health of mothers who likely suffered from kidney disease, hypertension (high blood pressure), heart disease, and diabetes. Mothers may also have been weak and prone to premature births and stillbirths because of poor diets, a common problem among mothers of the Yakama Nation in the early 20th century. Yakama mothers with any of these conditions were more likely to give birth prematurely and place the fetus in jeopardy.[73] Premature births could also be caused by spontaneous abortion, incompetent cervix, hydramnios, and premature rupture of membranes. Spontaneous abortion is commonly known as miscarriage, and it occurred when labor began before the 20th week of pregnancy. Premature births could develop when the fetus and placenta separated from the uterus, which could be brought on if one of the organs was defective or if the mother fell or was in an accident. In such cases, when the fetus was rejected before the 20th week of life, it usually died.[74]

Premature birth could also be caused by an incompetent cervix, a condition in which the cervix dilated early. Most often this occurred after the 14th week of pregnancy when the placenta and fetus detach from the inner uterus, causing a miscarriage. The cervix could be weak and unable to remain closed for nine months. In some cases the cervix could open early, delivering the baby prematurely. This kind of premature birth could also be caused by hydramnios, which was an accumulation of amniotic fluid inside the uterine wall. In most cases the accumulation of fluid was harmless, but in some cases, the uterus could swell with the fluid and labor could begin early. Although these cases were likely rare, they could occur, particularly if the mothers were diabetic, carrying two or more fetuses, or suffering from toxemia.

In addition to the causes mentioned above, premature birth could also develop if the membrane surrounding the baby ruptured. This was called "breaking water," and it was always part of the normal birthing process. In order for a delivery, the membranes had to burst, but if the membrane broke early, infection could develop before the baby was delivered. Early water breaking could endanger the life of the baby and mother. The rupture of the membrane surrounding the baby could also lead to premature birth, which, like infection, could endanger the baby's life.[75] Any of these causes of premature birth could have contributed to the premature delivery of fetuses on the Yakama Reservation. However, the actual causes of most miscarriages are unknown, because officials failed to provide detailed descriptions. On the Yakama Reservation, the descriptions provided in the death certificates generally stated that the cause of death was "prematurity," "premature development," or "premature birth." In a few descriptive cases, officials wrote that the death of an infant was caused by "immature birth," "hemorrhage premature," "premature with syphilis," "malnutrition and premature birth," and "premature birth sibling of [indicating the birth of twins]."[76]

Although stillbirth deaths of fetuses did not rank as one of the ten leading causes of death on the Yakama Reservation, it was the 13th leading cause of death in the general population and one of the two significant causes of fetal death. For this reason, it deserves attention. Medical professionals referred to stillbirth as intrauterine death of a fetus, and it occurred when a fetus was delivered after the 20th week of life. A mother suffering from toxemia or diabetes could contribute to the condition of delivering a stillborn baby. The condition could also be caused by a hemorrhage or an abnormality in the fetus.[77] Like premature births, "stillbirths are more common in poor communities, among older women, and when good prenatal and obstetric care is lacking."[78] Fetuses could be severely malformed and their condition could account for some stillbirths. A mother's health could also affect stillbirths, including hypertension, alcoholism, or antepartum hemorrhage. If the mother's placenta does not function correctly, a child could be born dead. This was particularly true if the child did not receive sufficient oxygen. A mother suffering from measles, rubella, herpes, syphilis, malaria, influenza, chickenpox, and other infectious diseases could also deliver a stillborn baby affected by a particular disease contracted from the mother.[79] All of these conditions could have caused stillbirths on the Yakama Reservation, although the death certificates and hospital records were silent on this point. Between 1888 and 1964, a large number of infants died of premature births (n = 64, or 61 percent) and stillbirths (n = 41, or 39 percent). Some of these conditions could have been prevented through childbirth education, prenatal care, and preventive medicine. The lack of medical care, attention, diet, and facilities was also a factor in the deaths of Yakama children.

Senility and Old Age

On the other end of the age spectrum, senility and old age accounted for the 10th leading cause of death on the Yakama Reservation (n = 57, or 3 percent), closely followed by strokes and alcohol-related deaths. Today, senility is described as "changes in mental ability caused by old age."[80] The condition is associated with loss of memory and concentration with the "risk of *dementia*, which affects about one in five of those over 80."[81] In the past, people used the term "senility" to describe old age, and county and state officials used the term in the Yakama death certificates as a common cause of death. In the early death certificates, recording officials noted this cause of death by writing that the person had died of "old age," "senility," or "inanition & debility-senility." Most often, officials designated this cause of death simply by stating that the person had died of senility, but this description was found primarily in those death certificates recorded between 1915 and 1932. After 1932, senility as a cause of death appeared only twice. People who died of this cause had likely lost control of their intellectual abilities and some may have suffered from dementia due to Alzheimer's disease, a loss of brain cells from certain parts of the brain. State and county recording agents may have also used the designation of senility to describe the elderly when officials did not know the exact cause of death. In any case, senility and old age accounted for 57 deaths on the Yakama Reservation.[82]

Year of Death

Year of death is a variable found on all the death certificates, and it is measured at an interval level. Death certificates nearly always provided the year of death, and so most of this data was complete since it was recorded regularly in the documents. The Yakama Agency collection contained a total of 3,899 death certificates, dealing with the years from 1888 to 1964. The data for the early years is incomplete. The Office of Indian Affairs reported only one death per year for the years from 1888 to 1901, and one death per year for the years 1908 and 1909. This was the lowest number of deaths per year recorded in the data set. The data between 1888 and 1910 is weak and does not represent accurately the number of deaths on the Yakama Reservation, but it is included with the other years because together the data offers insights into deaths for a lengthy period of time and into the neglect by the Office of Indian Affairs in recording vital statistics.

The highest number of recorded deaths occurred in 1928, when the agency recorded 229 deaths. In 1928, the government of the United States released the Meriam Report, and the large number of deaths recorded on the Yakama Reservation during this year was directly linked with the nationwide demand for better record keeping by the Indian Office, which was a major criticism by the entire study. Indeed, during the period from 1924 to 1941, government officials reported many more deaths on reservations, and agents preserved more death certificates on Yakama people than at any other time during the 76-year period under study. Between 1924 and 1941, they recorded and preserved a total of 2,323 deaths (60 percent) during the 17-year period. The Great Depression contributed to the large numbers of deaths, but the large number of deaths represented a reaction to national reforms in the Office of Indian Affairs and the leadership of John Collier as commissioner of Indian Affairs. In sum, the Indian Office began keeping vital statistics.

The number of Yakama recorded deaths declined dramatically during the 1940s, perhaps because of the decline in the number of deaths caused by tuberculosis, the isolation of tubercular cases, advancements in medicine, and the delivery of medicine on the reservation. The number of deaths also declined due to changes in the political world, which turned its attention to World War II and away from American Indian reforms. In any case, a major break in the epidemiological history of the Yakama developed in those years before and after the Second World War. The war was a pivotal watershed in Yakama history epidemiologically and nutritionally. After the war, far more Yakama people died of manmade diseases, while at the same time most Yakama turned to wage earning and cash payments that they used to buy manufactured foods. Fewer Yakama could hunt, fish, and gather as they had in the past, and the causes of death changed from contagious diseases to man-made problems such as heart disease, cancer, accidents, diabetes, and accidental deaths.

After World War II, the overall number of deaths on the Yakama Reservation declined significantly, and was due mainly to a decline in deaths caused by infectious diseases. The decline in overall deaths each year also resulted from better health care on the reservation and the introduction of an array of medicines, particularly antibiotics.[83] However, when anthropologist Eugene S. Hunn read this manuscript, he was "puzzled by the sharp drop in reported deaths after 1940." He noted that "while improved medical treatment and hygiene might account for some reduction, this is also a time when the total base population is growing rapidly, and in general, the larger the population, the more deaths."[84] Hunn is correct in pointing out that the drop in the numbers of deaths reported after 1940 may be attributed to the national preoccupation with the war and not recording accurate statistics. During the early 1940s, the United States turned its attention overseas, where the Second World War raged on many fronts. Washington officials working within the Office of Indian Affairs changed during this time period, and agency officials likely spent far less time collecting vital statistics on the reservations. Furthermore, qualified agency officials and employees left the agency to fight, and their replacements may not have been as committed to collecting vital statistics, which could account for the drop in overall deaths. However, the overall population living on the reservation may have declined as people moved to cities to work in war industries or enlisted in the armed services. While the agency added more names to the census rolls, the actual number of native residents on the reservation may have declined during the war years. The decline in the number of death certificates during the 1940s may have also been linked to changes in the federal government during the war and immediately afterward when the nation was more preoccupied with the spread of communism than the collection of vital statistics on Indian reservations. There may have been a change in reporting practices of the Yakama Agency after 1940 which, in part, accounts for the fewer number of reported deaths during the decade.[85]

Age at Death

The third variable coded in the study was the person's age at death, and county and state officials usually recorded the person's age on the death certificate. Between 1888 and 1964, the mean age of death on the Yakama Reservation was 33, with a standard deviation of five. For females, the mean age of death was 35, with a standard deviation of nine, and for males the mean age was 31, with a standard deviation of six and a half. We coded age at death as an interval-level variable from zero to ninety-nine, with zero representing the death of those children under one year of age and stillborn infants, and ninty-nine representing persons dying at ninety-nine years of age or older. Only a few individuals died at 99 years of age or older, and most of these were males. Importantly, the modal age of death was under one year of age, a circumstance common in many world populations. A total of 737, or 19 percent, of all deaths in the population from 1888 to 1964 occurred among Yakama fetuses and infants that died before one year of age. This was the largest number of deaths for any age group. Fetal deaths accounted for the demise of 106 fetuses (14 percent), and infant deaths accounted for the deaths of 631 infants (86 percent). A total of 235 children (6 percent) died between the age of one and two years of age, while 112 (3 percent) died between the ages of two and three. The number of deaths decreased as children got older, which was typical in human populations. A total of 67 (2 percent) children died during their third year, 62 (2 percent) during their fourth year, and 35 (1 percent) during their fifth year. Roughly one third of all deaths on the Yakama Reservation between 1888 and 1964 were those of children less than six years of age. The high number of infant and childhood deaths on the Yakama Reservation is similar to that found in some countries of Africa, Asia, and Latin America.

The distribution is skewed to the right due to the high number of deaths of infants and children under six years of age. A large number of deaths occurred among fetuses, infants, and children, and the Yakama people still lament the death of so many children.

Gender

Gender was the fourth variable in the study, measured as a nominal variable. Between 1888 and 1964, a total of 1,922 females (49 percent) died, while 1,960 males (50 percent) died, which is an even and normal split of the population. A total of 17 death certificates did not include the person's gender. The analysis of the data demonstrates that while females and males generally died of the same major causes of death, there were significant differences between male and female death rates for various causes. For example, Yakama females died in larger number from cancer, meningitis, stroke, natural causes, and childbirth, but none of these causes appear in the major causes of death among males. In the same way, premature birth and alcohol-related deaths were two of the foremost causes of death among Yakama males, but these two causes of death were not among the leading causes of death among females.

Place of Death

Place of death is a nominal variable, and the authors coded all deaths as occurring on the Yakama Reservation, off the reservation, or at unknown places. The authors determined the place of death in each case by consulting the place designated on the death certificate. For example, if the person died at Fort Simcoe, Toppenish, Harrah, White Swan, or Wapato, the authors coded them as having died on the reservation. If they died in Yakama City, Sunnyside, Moxee City, Spokane, Seattle, Portland, or Tacoma, the authors coded them as dying off the reservation. Thus, if the person died within the boundary lines of the reservation, we coded them as having died on the reservation, even though some of these individuals died in close proximity to the reservation and lived on the reservation. The authors did this in spite of the fact that traditional lands of Yakama Indians included more territory than those designated in the Yakama Treaty of 1855 and those lands recognized by the United States as the Yakama Reservation after allotment.[86]

The Yakama Reservation boundary lines changed over time and represented an artificial land division imposed on the Yakama Nation by the government. Such boundaries were nontraditional to Indian people, but they have been a part of Yakama history and the legal relationship between the Yakama Nation and the United States since the Senate ratified and the president signed the Yakama Treaty in 1859. For the purposes of this study, the authors used the boundaries of the reservation in spite of their shortcomings, simply to examine where deaths occurred. A total of 2,846 deaths (73 percent) occurred on the Yakama Reservation, while 932 deaths (24 percent) took place off the reservation. State officials did not report the place of death of 121 people (3 percent).

The authors examined the relationship between place of death and tribal affiliation (Yakama or non-Yakama), to determine if Yakama people generally died on their own reservation. Of the 2,846 Indians who died on the reservation, 2,164 (76 percent) were Yakama, 449 (16 percent) were non-Yakama (but most were identified tribally as among the people who were party to the Yakama Treaty of 1855), and 233 (8 percent) were not known. Of the 932 Native Americans who died off the Yakama Reservation, 391 (42 percent) were Yakama, 221 (24 percent) were non-Yakama, and 320 (34 percent) were not known. Yakama Indians died more often on their reservation than off the reservation and this is generally true of non-Yakama who were either visiting or living on the Yakama Reservation at the time of death. Often the non-Yakama came from tribes who were party to the Yakama treaty but who were non-Yakama or from other Northwestern reservations who were married or related to Yakama people. After an evaluation of this data, the authors determined it was not significant historically to warrant a further examination in the analysis of this work. While the data was interesting, it revealed little about Yakama deaths over time and little more than that which was mentioned above.

The fact that most deaths of Yakama Indians occurred on the reservation was likely due to the fact that the reservation was the land base and home of most Yakama Indians. They sometimes worked off the reservation and traveled to towns and other reservations, but since the reservation was home, they remained at home often, especially when they were ill. In addition, transportation systems were poor during much of the late 19th and early 20th centuries. Until the 1940s, few Yakama Indians died in truck and automobile accidents, but the 1940s witnessed the first major series of fatalities that occurred on and near the reservation. People sometimes visited reservation border towns to purchase groceries and other goods, but most people lived on the reservation. When individuals became ill, they remained home, particularly Indian people who received some medical care on their home reservation and could consult their own Indian doctors. Because of racial issues and the lack of money, Indians received little medical care off the reservation. Therefore, when individuals became ill, they tended to remain home, where they had familial support, traditional doctors, and some government medical care.

Conclusion

The statistics provided in this volume are not simply numbers. For the authors and for many American Indian people, they are the voices of the dead, the once living, breathing, vital people of the Yakama Indian Nation. When these people—nearly four thousand in number—passed away, their friends and relatives never thought of them as statistics. Contemporary native people of the great Columbia Plateau and coastal regions of Washington Idaho, British Columbia, and Oregon do not now think of the people presented in this work as mere statistics. The statistics they created by their dying provide us voices that speak to us over time and space. Through their dying, they inform us about life and death on one particular Indian reservation over a period of years. Through their deaths, the people tell us several stories, of which only a few appear in this presentation. It is our hope that other scholars will use these voices and tell more stories, historical accounts about the quality of life on the reservation during the early 20th century and change over time.

The death certificates from which this study is drawn survive as a collection in the National Archives, Pacific Northwest Region, on Sandpoint Way in Seattle, Washington. We made copies of over four thousand death certificates and used a total of 3,899 of them for this study, culling out repetitious certificates. After coding and quantifying all of the death certificates, we sent the documents to the Yakama Tribal Library in Toppenish, Washington, so that the people of the Yakama Nation could have access to their own records. Until a few years ago, the Yakama people did not have copies of these important documents, but now copies of all the certificates used in this study have found a new home in the heart of the Yakama Indian Reservation. For this presentation, we have included several of the documents, broken down by cause of death, year of death, age at death, gender, and place of death. However, we are still working through the documents dealing with automobile accidents, miscellaneous accidents, suicides, and murders, because we plan a future study to analyze these aspects of the data set. Most of our documents are contained herein, and they offer a rare window into life and death on the Yakama Indian Reservation through a statistical presentation of mortality over a period of time, primarily during the early to mid-20th century when officials of the Office of Indian Affairs and state of Washington kept the best records. We feel that our unique approach to the social history of the Yakama Reservation will entice other scholars to use these statistics to tell us more about conditions on the reservation, the diseases that killed so many people, and the tragedy of so many infant and childhood deaths.

We hope that readers will understand the many causes of death on the reservation and come to some appreciation of the battles that individuals, families, and communities fought just to stay alive in the wake of catastrophic changes. In addition to the implementation of the reservation system, the people had to live through an era of intense forced assimilation, loss of their children to boarding schools where some died, and destruction of their native economy. The loss of root grounds, berry fields, hunting areas, and fishing places proved dangerous and life-threatening to the people, as they lost access and use of their native foods. In addition to the loss of their nutritious native foods, the people lost their very close connection to this aspect of their daily and seasonal spiritual relationship with their foods, which all of them considered sacred and as part of their traditional religion. The people needed their foods for the biological and spiritual nourishment of their bodies, and when man-made conditions on the plateau prevented the people from consuming their native foods, their physical and mental health suffered severely. The loss of food did not cause tuberculosis, pneumonia, or influenza. Bacteria and viruses caused the diseases that took the lives of so many people. However, the loss of native foods contributed significantly to malnourishment among the people, and this contributed to their bodies' inability to effectively fight disease. The loss of native foods over time made people more vulnerable to disease and impaired their capacity to fight illnesses. In addition, although we cannot quantify this variable, we know that people suffered depression as a result of government policies that relegated a free people to confinement on reservations and the loss of thousands of acres of their former lands where they had prayed, hunted, fished, resided, conducted ceremonies, and gathered for generations.

The loss of native foods and their native lands provided a tragic and major epidemiological change for all the Indian people living on the Columbia Plateau, because the government did not replace native foods with foods sufficiently nutritious to stave off a fierce attack of bacteria and viruses that wracked the Yakama Nation and made the people more vulnerable to disease and death. The government of the United States, the territory and state of Washington, and white settlers created the circumstances that resulted in ill health, disease, and death on the Yakama Reservation. Malnutrition reigned on the reservations where children and adults, particularly pregnant mothers, suffered malnutrition. Government action and lack of action caused Indian families to turn to wage earning in order to survive. Wage earning resulted in people having less and less time to hunt, fish, and gather their native foods, and restriction of movement across their former domain resulted in illness and death. During the 20th century, many Yakama people continued to hunt, fish, and gather, at least to some degree, and some people in the 21st century continue to maintain those patterns. But in the 20th century, the traditional economy of Yakama people and their Plateau Indian neighbors no longer sustained them. As a result, the Yakama turned to labor on farms and ranches—a common development among Indians across the American West. The result of the government's takeover of Indian lands and their lives amounted to nothing less than genocide.

We believe that the statistical documentation found in this work supports the thesis that the government of the United States committed genocide against the people of the Yakama Nation. We base this on the definition of genocide offered in 1948 by the United Nations' "Convention on the Prevention and Punishment of the Crime of Genocide." Our study of Native American history in the Northwest leads us to assert that the government committed genocide against Yakama people by its "intent to destroy, in whole or in part, a national, ethnical, racial or religious group" by killing, causing bodily or mental harm, inflicting conditions calculated to bring about their physical destruction, imposing measures intended to prevent births, and forcibly transferring children of the group to another group.[87] The results of the physical invasion of Yakama people, forced removal and establishment of the reservation system, removal of children from their parents to boarding schools, destruction of native food resources, and medical neglect of the people during much of the reservation era resulted in a domestic genocide.

Yakama people survived, but contemporary descendents still deal with the ill effects of government policies of the 19th and 20th centuries. The reservation proved an unhealthy place for Yakama people. They suffered many illnesses and deaths as demonstrated by the statistics found here. But the Yakama people overcame many of the adversities created by the government. They survived a horrific biological attack of bacteria and viruses that took the lives of so many of their people. Contemporary tribal people living on and off the Yakama Reservation are descendents of a tenacious people whose voices ring clear through the statistics presented in this study. They suffered greatly from disease and death, but they survived to tell this story through the act of their own dying.

Notes

1. See Helen H. Schuster, *The Yakima*, Indians of North America Series, ed. Frank W. Porter III (New York: Chelsea House Publishers, 1990), 21–22.

2. Donald W. Meinig, *The Great Columbia Plain: A Historical Geography, 1805–1910* (Seattle: University of Washington Press, 1968).

3. Schuster, *The Yakima*, 21–24, and Clifford E. Trafzer, *Death Stalks the Yakama: Epidemiological Transitions and Mortality on the Yakama Indian Reservation, 1888–1964* (East Lansing: Michigan State University Press, 1997), 25–27.

4. Oral interview with Mary Jim, April 25, 1980, Yakama Indian Reservation, Trafzer personal collection.

5. Oral interview with Mary Jim, April 25, 1980.

6. Oral interview with Mary Jim, April 25, 1980.

7. Trafzer, *Death Stalks the Yakama*, 32–33.

8. For discussions of the arrival of epidemics on the Columbia Plateau, see Meinig, *The Great Columbia Plain*; Robert T. Boyd, "Introduction of Infectious Diseases among the Indians of the Pacific Northwest, 1774–1874" (PhD diss., University of Washington, 1975); and Eugene Hunn with James Selam and family, *Nch'i-Wana "The Big River": Mid-Columbia Indians and Their Land* (Seattle: University of Washington Press, 1990).

9. Robert R. McCoy, *Chief Joseph, Yellow Wolf, and the Creation of Nez Perce History in the Pacific Northwest* (New York: Routledge Press, 2004), 73–76.

10. The best discussions of the war are in Alvin M. Josephy, Jr., *The Nez Perce Indians and the Opening of the Northwest*, abridged ed. (Lincoln: University of Nebraska Press, 1971), 324–76, and Clifford E. Trafzer and Richard D. Scheuerman, *Renegade Tribe: The Palouse Indians and the Invasion of the Inland Pacific Northwest* (Pullman: Washington State University Press, 1986), 60–92.

11. The best general discussion of assimilation efforts and the Dawes Act is found in Frederick E. Hoxie, *A Final Promise: The Campaign to Assimilate the Indians, 1880–1920* (Lincoln: University of Nebraska Press, 1989).

12. Schuster, *The Yakima*, 80–84.

13. Available at http://www.ccrh.org/comm/primary/yaktreaty.html.

14. For a thorough examination of the historical literature of the Yakama and other Sahaptin-speaking Indians of the Northwest, see Clifford E. Trafzer, *Yakima, Palouse, Cayuse, Umatilla, Walla Walla, and Wanapum Indians: An Historical Bibliography* (Metuchen, N.J.: Scarecrow Press, 1991).

15. Abdel R. Omran, "Epidemiologic Transition in the United States: The Health Factor in Population Change," *Population Bulletin* 32 (1977): 16–18.

16. The finest scholarly work on the topic is Boyd, "Introduction of Infectious Disease among the Indians of the Pacific Northwest, 1774–1874."

17. Barry M. Popkin, "Nutritional Patterns and Transitions," *Population and Development Review* 19 (1993): 138–45.

18. Samuel H. Preston and Michael R. Haines, *Fatal Years: Child Mortality in Late Nineteenth-Century America* (Princeton, N.J.: Princeton University Press, 1991), 171; George Alter, "Infant and Child Mortality in the United States," paper prepared for "La Mortalite des Enfants dans le Passe," *International Union for the Scientific Study of Population*, University of Montreal (October 7–9, 1992): 6–7.

19. John R. Weeks to Clifford E. Trafzer, June 15, 1994, author's collection.

20. Weeks to Trafzer, June 15, 1994.

21. Weeks to Trafzer, June 15, 1994.

22. Edward D. Castillo, "The Impact of Euro-American Exploration and Settlement," *Handbook of North American Indians*, ed. Robert F. Heizer (Washington, D.C.: Smithsonian Institution Press, 1978), 118, 123, 124; Keith H. Basso, 'Western Apache," *Handbook of North American Indians Southwest* (Washington, D.C.: Smithsonian Institution Press, 1983); and Robert L. Bergman, "Navajo Health Services and Projects," *Southwest*, ed. Alfonso Ortiz (Washington, D.C.: Smithsonian Institution Press, 1983), 482–83, 672–77; Clifford E. Trafzer and Richard D. Scheuerman, *Chief Joseph's Allies* (Newcastle, Calif.: Sierra Oaks Publishing Company, 1992); 83–87; Russell Thornton, *American Indian Holocaust and Survival: A Population History Since 1492* (Norman: University of Oklahoma Press, 1987), 99–104, 125–27.

23. *Puyallup Tribe v. Department of Game*, Supreme Court of the United States, 1968, 391 United States 392, 88 Supreme Court 1725. 20 L. Ed. 2nd 689, in David H. Getches and Charles F. Wilkinson, *Federal Indian Law* (St. Paul, Minn.: West Publishing Company, 1986), 734–40. The law discussed in this case is applied to the Yakama and appeared in the 1969 case *Sohappy v. Smith* and the 1974 case *United States v. Washington.*

24. Charles J. Kappler, *Indian Affairs, Laws, and Treaties, 2 Volumes* (Washington, D.C.: Government Printing Office, 1940), 698–702; *Documents Relating to Negotiations of Ratified and Unratified Treaties of the United States*, NA, RG 75, Microfilm T494, Reel 5. During the treaty negotiations at the Walla Walla Council, Stevens specifically guaranteed the Yakama and others the continued right to fish, hunt, and gather wherever they had done so in the past, both on and off the reservation.

25. Clifford E. Trafzer and Margery Ann Beach, "Smohalla, the Washani, and Religion as a Factor in Northwestern Indian History," *American Indian Quarterly* 9 (1985): 73, 75–77. Although Plateau Indians had acquired seeds from Hudson's Bay

Company traders and had planted gardens, they continued to maintain their traditional economic life. During the early reservation era, some of the people ranched and farmed, but most continued traditional seasonal rounds. Yet, with the destruction of the root grounds, salmon, and game, Indians turned to ranching and farming. See Schuster, "Yakima Indian Traditionalism," 204, 238, 262. For destruction of salmon through irrigation projects, see Yakima Tribal Council, *The Yakimas: Treaty Centennial, 1855–1955* (Yakima, Wash.: Republic Press, 1955), 36, 48. The dams in the Northwest also destroyed the salmon runs. See these general studies on dams located on the Columbia River and its tributaries: United States Department of the Army, *Review Report on Columbia River and Tributaries*, Corps of Engineers, North Pacific Division, October 1, 1948; United States Department of Interior, "The Columbia River," *House Executive Document* 473, 81st Congress, 2nd Session 1950; Bureau of Indian Affairs, *Report on the Source, Nature and Extent of the Fishing, Hunting and Miscellaneous Related Rights of Certain Tribes in Washington and Oregon* (Los Angeles: Office of Indian Affairs, Division of Forestry and Grazing, 1942); and T. W. Mermel, ed. and comp., *Register of Dams in the United States: Completed, Under Construction and Proposed* (New York: McGraw Hill, 1958).

26. Schuster, *The Yakama*, 29–30.

27. L. V. McWhorter, *The Crime Against the Yakima* (North Yakima, Wash.: Republic Press, 1913). McWhorter reported that the Yakama lived in one- or two-room shacks with lean-to kitchens. Also see Schuster, "Yakima Indian Traditionalism," 68–87.

28. Omran, "Epidemiologic Transition in the United States," 8, 9, 18.

29. Schuster, 'Yakima Indian Traditionalism," 165–76.

30. Trafzer and Scheuerman, *Renegade Tribe*, 26; S. F. Cook, "The Epidemic of 1830–33 in California and Oregon," *University of California Publications in Archaeology and Ethnology* 43 (1955): 303–26; Thornton, *American Indian Holocaust*, 99.

31. Yakama Death Certificates, NA, PNWR, RG 75. Many unknown cases can be cited, including 4537, 4540, 4541, 4542, 4543, 4552, 4558. The author chose not to disclose the name of any person found on the death certificates in order to protect the privacy of Yakama families.

32. Diane T. Putney, "Robert Grosvenor Valentine, 1909–1912," in *The Commissioners of Indian Affairs*, ed. Robert M. Kvasnicka and Herman J. Viola (Lincoln: University of Nebraska Press, 1979), 233–42. Putney has also written an outstanding scholarly work on Indian health from 1900 to 1930. See Diane T. Putney, "Fighting the Scourge: American Indian Morbidity and Federal Policy, 1897–1928" (PhD diss., Marquette University, 1980).

33. Schuster, "Yakima Indian Traditionalism," 80–83. Allotment of the Yakama Reservation ended in 1914, with 4,506 Yakama people securing for themselves 440,000 acres of individual allotments and 780,000 of tribally owned land. In 1992, the Yakama owned 253,280 acres of the original 440,000 acres, and most of the best farmland with water had been purchased by non-Indians.

34. Scholars should take note of the excellent work recently completed by Todd Benson of Stanford University on the health care of Native Americans during the early 20th century before the Public Health Service took over Indian health care.

Benson has conducted the most in-depth research on the topic. See Todd Benson, "Race, Health, and Power: The Federal Government and American Indian Health, 1909–1955" (PhD diss., Stanford University, 1993).

35. Lawrence C. Kelly, "Charles Henry Burke, 1921–29" and "Charles James Rhoads, 1929–33," and Kenneth R. Philp, "John Collier, 1933–45," in *The Commissioners of Indian Affairs*, ed. Robert M. Kvasnicka and Herman J. Viola (Lincoln: University of Nebraska Press, 1979), 253, 255, 268, 277. The author will provide further analysis of crude death rate, but briefly, the evidence is overwhelming that the agents on the Yakama Reservation did not record any infant deaths. In a comparison of death rates, the rates on the reservation are markedly lower than those for the United States as per thousand in the population. For example, in 1920, the U.S. crude death rate was ten to one when compared with the death rate on the Yakama Reservation. However, birth records are available for the Yakama from 1926 through 1931, and an infant mortality rate is calculated in the analysis, which demonstrates the high rate of infant mortality.

36. Lewis Meriam, *The Problem of Indian Administration* (New York: Johnson Reprint Corporation, 1971), 170–82.

37. Meriam, *The Problem of Indian Administration*, 189.

38. Meriam, *The Problem of Indian Administration*, 189.

39. Meriam, *The Problem of Indian Administration*, 189.

40. Meriam, *The Problem of Indian Administration*, 266.

41. Meriam, *The Problem of Indian Administration*, 266.

42. Meriam, *The Problem of Indian Administration*, 266.

43. H. De Lien and J. Nixon Hadley, "How to Recognize an Indian Health Problem," *Human Organization* (1952): 33.

44. De Lien and Hadley, "How to Recognize an Indian Health Problem," 33.

45. De Lien and Hadley, "How to Recognize an Indian Health Problem," 33.

46. Yakama Indian Census, 1885–1931, PNWR, NA, RG 75, Seattle, Washington.

47. Yakama Death Certificates, 1888 to 1910, NA, PNWR, RG 75.

48. No attempt is made to compare the death certificates of the Yakama Reservation with any other reservation since no database exists to do so, except the original death certificates for other reservations in the National Archives. The author plans to collect and analyze some of these documents in the future and use them to compare with the Yakama data.

49. Trafzer and Scheuerman, *Renegade Tribe*, 25–26; Robert H. Ruby and John A. Brown, *The Cayuse Indians* (Norman: University of Oklahoma Press, 1972), 103–8; Clifford E. Trafzer, *The Chinook* (New York: Chelsea House Publishers, 1990), 34–35. The best work on disease among Northwestern tribes is Boyd, "The Introduction of Infectious Diseases among the Indians of the Pacific Northwest, 1774–1874," 81–90, 99–100, 112–45, and 338–50. Also see Hunn, *Nch'i-Wana*, 27–32, 241.

50. Omran, "Epidemiologic Transition in the United States," 16.

51. Yakama Death Certificates, NA, PNWR, RG 75, Cases 4795, 462, 2768, 1203, 206, 2958, 489, 696, 3462, 3565.

52. Yakama Death Certificates, NA, PNWR, RG 75, Case 1160; Jeffrey R. M. Kunz and Asher J. Finkel, *The American Medical Association Family Medical Guide* (New York: Random House, 1987), 574, 719, 748; Wesley W. Spink, *Infectious Diseases: Pre-*

vention and Treatment in Nineteenth and Twentieth Centuries (Minneapolis: University of Minnesota Press, 1978), 209–12; Ales Hrdlickas, "Tuberculosis among Certain Indian Tribes in the United States," *Annual Report of the Bureau of American Ethnography* 42 (Washington, D.C.: Smithsonian Institution, 1909), 32–32; Spink, *Infectious Diseases*, 220–21, 224; Frank McFarlan Bumet and David O. White, *Natural History of Infectious Diseases* (Cambridge: Cambridge University Press, 1972), 213–24; Jay Arthur Meyers, *Captain of All These Men of Death* (St. Louis, Mo.: Warren H. Green, 1977), 73–83, 142–58; Selman A. Waksman, *The Conquest of Tuberculosis* (Berkeley: University of California Press, 1964), 24, 204–8. The most penetrating and significant work on the subject in recent years is Barbara Bates, *Bargaining for Life: A Social History of Tuberculosis, 1876–1938* (Philadelphia: University of Pennsylvania Press, 1992).

53. Yakama Death Certificates, NA, PNWR, RG 75, Cases 179, 202, 701, 2837, 3031.

54. Charles B. Clayman, ed., *The American Medical Association Encyclopedia of Medicine* (New York: Random House, 1989), 803.

55. Spink, *Infectious Diseases*, 209–12; Bumet and White, *Natural History of Infectious Diseases*, 32–43, 52–69; Andrew B. Christie, *Infectious Diseases: Epidemiology and Clinical Practice* (Edinburgh and London: E. and S. Livingstone, 1969), 269–99; and Kunz and Finkel, *Family Medical Guide*, 365–695. For general medical studies, specifically on pneumonia, see William S. Lynn, ed., *Inflammatory Cells and Lung Disease* (Boca Raton, Fla.: CRC Press, 1983); James E. Pennington, ed., *Respiratory Infections: Diagnosis and Management* (New York: Raven Press, 1983); Selwyn DeWitt Collins and Josephine Lehmann, *Excess Deaths from Influenza and Pneumonia and from Important Chronic Diseases during Epidemic Periods, 1918–1951* (Washington, D.C.: Public Health Service, 1953).

56. John R. Weeks to Clifford E. Trafzer, June 15, 1994, Trafzer personal collection.

57. Clayton, ed., *Encyclopedia of Medicine*, 803.

58. Oral discussion, February 17, 1995, University of California, Berkeley.

59. Yakama Death Certificates, NA, PNWR, RG 75, Cases 2445, 231, 476, 697.

60. Popkin, "Nutritional Patterns and Transitions," 138–46.

61. Omran, "Epidemiologic Transition in the United States," 17.

62. Kunz and Finkle, *Family Medical Guide*, 380–86.

63. Kunz and Finkle, *Family Medical Guide*, 388, 640.

64. Yakama Death Certificates, NA, PNWR, RG 75, Cases 118, 49, 588, 3203, 3402, 3789, 3835, 2933, 70, 336, 94, 597, 9930, 2387, 2839, 3486, 3872, 3494.

65. Kunz and Finkle, *Family Medical Guide*, 467, 664, 702; Christie, *Infectious Diseases*, 122–67; Spink, *Infectious Diseases*, 246–47; Burnet and White, *Natural History of Infectious Diseases*, 70–87. For general medical works on gastrointestinal disorders, see Marvin H. Sleisenger and John S. Fordtran, eds., *Gastrointestinal Disease* (Philadelphia: W.B. Saunders, 1989); Emanuel Lebenthan, ed., *Textbook of Gastroenterology and Nutrition in Infancy* (New York: Raven Press, 1981); and S. C. Truelove, *Diseases of the Digestive System* (Oxford: Blackwell Scientific Publications, 1972). Another form of gastrointestinal disorder is caused by a viral infection from food and liquid, although this is rare.

66. Yakama Death Certificates, NA, PNWR, RG 75, Cases 478, 611, 865, 1293, 2427, 2696, 4510.

67. Kunz and Finkle, *Family Medical Guide*, 570–71, 365.

68. Yakama Death Certificates, NA, PNWR, RG 75, Cases 9245, 247, 2402, 3984, 3989, 246, 338, 1145, 1287.

69. Trafzer, *The Chinook*, 34–35.

70. Yakama Death Certificates, NA, PNWR, RG 75, Cases 536, 605, 1236, 2429, 3189, 3463, 3510, 3584, 3791, 3847, 4001, 4517, 4417.

71. According to Brad Richie, M.D., and Professor James Sandos, University of Redlands, doctors could not distinguish between uterine and cervical cancers without conducting autopsies. It is unlikely that many autopsies, if any, were performed on these women. Sandos suggested that the two types of cancer would be more properly labeled venereal cancer.

72. Kunz and Finkle, *Family Medical Guide*, 47, 711.

73. Clayton, ed., *Encyclopedia of Medicine*, 817.

74. Kunz and Finkle, *Family Medical Guide*, 643–48; Wenda R. Trevathan, *Human Birth: An Evolutionary Perspective* (New York: Aldine de Gruyter, 1987), 12, 21, 67, 93, 98, 119, 124–25, 141–42, 199, 228. For medical studies on premature births, see Beryl Dorothy Comer, *Prematurity: The Diagnosis, Care and Disorders of the Premature Infant* (London: Cassell, 1960); Julius H. Hess and Evelyn C. Lundeen, *The Premature Infant* (Philadelphia: Lippincott, 1949); and Evelyn C. Lundeen and Ralph H. Kunstadter, *Care of the Premature Infant* (Philadelphia: Lippincott, 1958). Most of the medical works on premature births deal with the medical problems of dealing with the child that survives, and they do not analyze the issue of high infant mortality resulting from premature births. The 20th week is counted from the first day of the last period.

75. Kunz and Finkle, *Family Medical Guide*, 643–48.

76. Yakama Death Certificates, NA, PNWR, RG 75, Cases 4179, 4165, 4384, 878, 699, 3206, 4381, 2377, 2878.

77. Trevathan, *Human Birth*, 11–12, 21, 75, 105, 142; Kunz and Finkle, *Family Medical Guide*, 647.

78. Clayton, ed., *Encyclopedia of Medicine*, 941.

79. Clayton, ed., *Encyclopedia of Medicine*, 941.

80. Clayton, ed., *Encyclopedia of Medicine*, 891.

81. Clayton, ed., *Encyclopedia of Medicine*, 891.

82. Yakama Death Certificates, NA, PNWR, RG 75, Cases 120, 4314; Kunz and Finkle, *Family Medical Guide*, 742.

83. Meriam, *The Problem of Indian Administration*, 189–345; Kenneth R. Philp, *John Collier's Crusade for Indian Reform, 1920–1954* (Tucson: University of Arizona Press, 1977), 114, 126–27, 130, 134.

84. Hunn to Trafzer, May 18, 1994.

85. Hunn to Trafzer, May 18, 1994.

86. Kappler, *Indian Law*, 698–702.

87. United Nations Convention on the Prevention and Punishment of the Crime of Genocide, available at http://www.hrweb.org/legal/genocide.html.

Tuberculosis

Mycobacteria Tuberculosis is an ancient disease, found in the bones and tissue of mummified bodies of Africa, Europe, Asia, and the Americas. It is an old disease, but it did not become a major killer of people until humans began living in concentrated areas. As a result of major changes brought on by trade, immigration, unit housing, and nutrition, tuberculosis spread as a killer among people. American Indian people suffered little from tuberculosis until their bodies became more susceptible to the disease due to stress, concentrated housing, and the lack of native foods. Tuberculosis spread rapidly in virgin populations, particularly after the United States created the reservation system. Yakama people had once lived in small villages along the river systems of the Inland Northwest, but the invasion of American troops and the creation of the Yakama Reservation in 1855 brought about the changes that proved conducive to tuberculosis. After the Plateau Indian Wars of the 1850s, the United States forced thousands of Indians onto reservations, concentrating many diverse tribal people in smaller areas where they could no longer live in traditional ways.

The government created the Yakama Reservation in 1855, forcing several different tribal peoples onto relatively small parcels of land where most lived in one-room makeshift houses with dirt floors and poor ventilation. Confined more and more to the reservation, non-Indians came into greater contact with Indian people working for the Office of Indian Affairs, Army, and railroads. White farmers and ranchers moved onto lands adjacent to the reservation, and non-Indian health seekers soon found their way into the Yakima Valley, looking for a cure for tuberculosis. They camped in tents or lived in crude dwellings to take in the clean, cool air and drink the clear, cold waters of the streams and rivers flowing across or near Indian lands. Owners of health resorts hired Indians to cook, clean rooms, wash infected sheets and blankets, and to tend those infected with tuberculosis. This close contact contributed to the spread of tuberculosis among Indian people.

Tuberculosis and scrofula, a glandular form of the disease, usually spread through the air but could also be passed from hand to mouth. The bacteria generally traveled through the air in tiny droplets, attaching to dust particles that unsuspecting people breathed into their lungs. However, the bacillus lived everywhere, including the soil and within birds, cattle, and other animals. It lived in the blood and phlegm emitted from nasty coughs of those infected with the disease, and it lived in the oozing pus left on handkerchiefs, pillowcases, clothing, and bedding of tuberculars. When people slept with tuberculars, drank from the same cups, or handled infected cloth, pipes, or musical instruments, they could easily contract the disease. When the bacilli entered the body, the immune system walled off the bacteria. In healthy bodies, the immune system could contain the bacillus, but in bodies weakened from malnutrition, stress, and secondary infections, the tubercle bacillus spread—sometimes rapidly killing the person without the typical long-term symptoms of the disease such as a bloody cough, loss of weight, weakness, fever, anemia, bone disease, meningitis, and arthritis. This was particularly true of Yakama infants and babies exposed to the disease and dying of a respiratory illness, which agents often identified in the death certificates as pneumonia, not tuberculosis. When tuberculosis invaded the bodies of babies, the bacteria found a vulnerable host with a weakened or impaired immune system unable to fight off the infection.

Between 1888 and 1964, tuberculosis reigned as the foremost killer of Yakama people, constituting nearly 30 percent of all deaths found on the reservation during this era. Furthermore, deaths caused by the disease declined in the 1940s and became negligible after 1950. No doubt antibiotics and health care that emphasized the isolation of tubercular patients to the Indian sanatorium located at Fort Lapwai on the Nez Perce Reservation of Idaho contributed to the decline of deaths. Furthermore, throughout the 20th century, Indian people learned a great deal about the "white plague," its causes, and prevention. Indians shared information about the disease, especially children returning home from schools where non-Indians taught hygiene, sanitation, and the budding field of public health. Thus, Indian agency played prominently into the decline of tuberculosis on the Yakama Reservation, but by the 1940s, the disease had begun to play out because of the use of antibiotics. In 1943, Selman Waksman, an American bacteriologist, discovered that streptomycin extracted from a mold proved effective against tuberculosis—a key component today in pharmaceutical cocktails used to fight tuberculosis. In 1947, American doctors began using streptomycin, but found that it could be toxic. In 1952, scientists began using isoniazid or INH, which became the primary antibiotic against tuberculosis. This disease among the Indian people living on the Yakama Reservation declined during the 1940s, but its legacy remains a dreaded subject in the memories of Indian people throughout the Northwest and in the documents preserved in the National Archives and offered here in this volume.

Year	Age	Gender	Place	Explanation
1911	40	F	Yakama	Tuberculosis
1911	48	F	Yakama	Pulmonary Tuberculosis
1915	75	F	Yakama	Tuberculosis
1915	36	M	Yakama	Tuberculosis
1915	49	F	Yakama	Tuberculosis
1916	39	M	Yakama	Tuberculosis
1916	24	M	Yakama	Tuberculosis
1916	13	M	Yakama	Tuberculosis
1916	50	F	Yakama	Tuberculosis
1916	45	F	Yakama	Tuberculosis
1916	17	F	Yakama	Tuberculosis
1916	40	M	Yakama	Tuberculosis
1917	7	F	Yakama	Pulmonary Tuberculosis
1917	1	F	Yakama	Pulmonary Tuberculosis
1917	13	F	Yakama	Pulmonary Tuberculosis
1917	1	F	Yakama	Pulmonary Tuberculosis
1917	10	F	Yakama	Pulmonary Tuberculosis
1917	7	F	Yakama	Pulmonary Tuberculosis
1917	39	M	Yakama	Pulmonary Tuberculosis
1917	38	F	Yakama	Pulmonary Tuberculosis
1917	57	F	Yakama	Pulmonary Tuberculosis
1917	1	M	Yakama	Pulmonary Tuberculosis
1917	1	F	Yakama	Pulmonary Tuberculosis
1917	6	F	Yakama	Pulmonary Tuberculosis
1918	6	M	Yakama	Tuberculosis of Bones
1918	66	F	Yakama	Pulmonary Tuberculosis
1918	4	F	Yakama	Pulmonary Tuberculosis
1918	24	F	Yakama	Pulmonary Tuberculosis
1918	1	F	Yakama	Pulmonary Tuberculosis
1918	1	F	Yakama	Pulmonary Tuberculosis
1918	4	F	Yakama	Tuberculosis
1918	1	M	Yakama	Tuberculosis
1918	16	M	Yakama	Tuberculosis
1918	14	F	Yakama	Tuberculosis
1918	9	M	Yakama	Tuberculosis
1918	73	F	Yakama	Tuberculosis
1918	1	F	Yakama	Tuberculosis
1919	26	M	Yakama	Tuberculosis
1919	17	M	Yakama	Tuberculosis
1919	1	M	Yakama	Tuberculosis

Year	Age	Gender	Place	Explanation
1920	17	F	Yakama	Tuberculosis
1922	18	F	Yakama	Tuberculosis
1922	13	F	Yakama	Tuberculosis
1924	74	F	Yakama	Pulmonary Tuberculosis
1924	54	F	Yakama	Tuberculosis
1924	27	F	Yakama	Pulmonary Tuberculosis
1924	16	F	Yakama	Tuberculosis
1924	11	M	Yakama	Tuberculosis
1924	15	M	Yakama	Tuberculosis
1924	14	M	Yakama	Tuberculosis
1924	19	M	Yakama	Tuberculosis
1924	8	F	Yakama	Tuberculosis
1924	6	F	Yakama	Tuberculosis
1924	57	F	Yakama	Tuberculosis
1924	33	M	Yakama	Tuberculosis
1924	11	M	Yakama	Tuberculosis
1924	7	F	Yakama	Tuberculosis
1924	6	F	Yakama	Tuberculosis
1924	50	F	Yakama	Tuberculosis
1924	19	F	Yakama	Tuberculosis
1924	57	F	Yakama	Tuberculosis
1924	37	M	Yakama	Tuberculosis
1925	59	F	Yakama	Tuberculosis
1925	67	F	Yakama	Tuberculosis
1925	34	F	Yakama	Tuberculosis
1925	18	F	Yakama	Tuberculosis
1925	23	M	Yakama	Tuberculosis
1925	22	M	Yakama	General Tuberculosis
1925	11	F	Yakama	Tuberculosis
1925	45	F	Yakama	Tuberculosis
1925	38	F	Yakama	Tuberculosis
1925	60	M	Yakama	Pulmonary Tuberculosis
1925	17	F	Yakama	Tuberculosis
1925	61	F	Yakama	Tuberculosis
1925	44	M	Yakama	Tuberculosis
1925	18	F	Yakama	Tuberculosis
1925	12	M	Yakama	Tuberculosis
1925	2	M	Yakama	Pulmonary Tuberculosis
1925	25	M	Yakama	Tuberculosis
1925	12	M	Yakama	Tuberculosis

Year	Age	Gender	Place	Explanation
1925	80	M	Yakama	Tuberculosis
1925	11	M	Yakama	Tuberculosis
1925	15	M	Yakama	Tuberculosis
1925	9	M	Off Rez	Tuberculosis
1925	25	M	Yakama	Tuberculosis
1925	44	M	Yakama	Tuberculosis
1925	51	M	Yakama	Tuberculosis
1925	60	M	Yakama	Tuberculosis
1925	12	M	Yakama	Tuberculosis
1926	38	F	Yakama	Tuberculosis
1926	2	F	Yakama	Tuberculosis
1926	26	F	Yakama	Tuberculosis
1926	35	F	Yakama	Tuberculosis
1926	23	M	Yakama	Tuberculosis
1926	23	F	Yakama	Tuberculosis
1926	14	M	Yakama	Tuberculosis
1926	39	F	Yakama	Tuberculosis
1926	69	F	Yakama	Tuberculosis
1926	22	M	Yakama	Tuberculosis
1926	39	F	Yakama	Pulmonary Tuberculosis
1926	6	F	Yakama	Glandular Tuberculosis
1926	65	F	Yakama	Tuberculosis
1926	8	F	Yakama	Tuberculosis
1926	2	F	Yakama	Tuberculosis
1926	14	M	Yakama	Tuberculosis
1926	14	M	Yakama	Tuberculosis
1926	26	F	Yakama	Pulmonary Tuberculosis
1926	21	M	Yakama	Pulmonary Tuberculosis
1926	24	M	Yakama	Tuberculosis
1926	56	M	Yakama	Tuberculosis
1926	24	M	Yakama	Tuberculosis
1926	42	F	Yakama	Tuberculosis
1926	20	M	Yakama	Tuberculosis
1926	56	M	Yakama	Tuberculosis
1926	18	M	Yakama	Tuberculosis
1927	17	M	Yakama	Tuberculosis
1927	3	M	Yakama	Tuberculosis
1927	76	F	Yakama	Tuberculosis
1927	18	M	Yakama	Tuberculosis
1927	24	M	Yakama	Tuberculosis

Year	Age	Gender	Place	Explanation
1927	25	F	Yakama	Tuberculosis
1927	9	M	Yakama	Tuberculosis
1927	28	F	Yakama	Tuberculosis
1927	50	F	Yakama	Tuberculosis
1927	71	M	Yakama	Tuberculosis
1927	17	F	Yakama	Tuberculosis
1927	21	M	Yakama	Tuberculosis
1927	76	F	Yakama	Tuberculosis
1927	43	M	Yakama	Pulmonary Tuberculosis
1927	23	M	Yakama	Tuberculosis
1927	17	F	Yakama	Tuberculosis
1927	10	M	Yakama	Pulmonary Tuberculosis
1927	10	M	Yakama	Pulmonary Tuberculosis
1927	15	F	Yakama	Pulmonary Tuberculosis
1927	50	F	Yakama	Tuberculosis
1927	19	M	Yakama	Tuberculosis
1927	33	F	Yakama	Tuberculosis
1927	32	F	Yakama	Tuberculosis
1927	32	F	Yakama	Tuberculosis
1927	8	M	Yakama	Tuberculosis
1927	7	F	Yakama	Tuberculosis
1927	61	F	Yakama	Tuberculosis
1927	15	F	Yakama	Tuberculosis
1927	65	F	Off Rez	Tuberculosis
1927	65	F	Yakama	Tuberculosis
1927	33	F	Yakama	Tuberculosis
1927	43	M	Yakama	Tuberculosis
1928	18	F	Yakama	Tuberculosis
1928	26	F	Yakama	Tuberculosis
1928	7	M	Yakama	Tuberculosis
1928	3	F	Yakama	Tuberculosis
1928	64	M	Off Rez	Tuberculosis
1928	24	M	Yakama	Tuberculosis
1928	12	F	Yakama	Pulmonary Tuberculosis
1928	52	M	Yakama	Tuberculosis
1928	21	M	Yakama	Pulmonary Tuberculosis
1928	27	F	Yakama	Tuberculosis
1928	26	F	Yakama	Pulmonary Tuberculosis
1928	7	M	Yakama	Pulmonary Tuberculosis
1928	24	M	Yakama	Tuberculosis

Year	Age	Gender	Place	Explanation
1928	31	M	Yakama	Tuberculosis
1928	12	M	Yakama	Tuberculosis
1928	12	F	Yakama	Pulmonary Tuberculosis
1928	16	F	Yakama	Pulmonary Tuberculosis
1928	38	F	Yakama	Tuberculosis
1928	6	M	Yakama	Pulmonary Tuberculosis
1928	0	F	Yakama	Tuberculosis
1928	48	F	Yakama	Tuberculosis
1928	22	M	Yakama	Pulmonary Tuberculosis
1928	24	F	Off Rez	—
1928	43	F	Yakama	—
1928	57	F	Yakama	—
1928	64	M	Yakama	—
1928	57	M	Yakama	—
1928	8	F	Yakama	—
1928	28	M	Yakama	—
1928	22	M	Yakama	—
1928	5	M	Yakama	—
1928	28	F	Yakama	—
1928	5	F	Yakama	—
1928	14	F	Yakama	—
1928	1	M	Yakama	—
1928	20	F	Off Rez	Tuberculosis
1928	0	M	Off Rez	Tuberculosis
1928	0	F	Yakama	Tuberculosis
1928	50	M	Off Rez	Tuberculosis
1928	10	M	Off Rez	Tuberculosis
1928	11	F	Off Rez	Tuberculosis
1928	11	F	Yakama	Tuberculosis
1928	5	M	Yakama	Tuberculosis
1928	2	F	Off Rez	Tuberculosis
1928	12	M	Off Rez	Tuberculosis
1928	41	M	Off Rez	Tuberculosis
1928	42	F	Off Rez	Tuberculosis
1928	87	M	Off Rez	Tuberculosis
1928	12	F	Off Rez	Tuberculosis
1928	29	F	Off Rez	Tuberculosis
1928	25	M	Off Rez	Tuberculosis
1928	5	F	Off Rez	Tuberculosis
1928	10	M	Off Rez	Tuberculosis

Year	Age	Gender	Place	Explanation
1928	0	M	Off Rez	Tuberculosis
1929	5	M	Yakama	—
1929	14	F	Yakama	—
1929	48	M	Yakama	—
1929	48	F	Yakama	—
1929	21	F	Yakama	—
1929	22	F	Yakama	Pulmonary Tuberculosis
1929	21	F	Yakama	Consumption
1929	5	M	Yakama	Tuberculosis
1929	14	F	Yakama	Pulmonary Tuberculosis
1929	14	F	Yakama	Tuberculosis
1929	0	F	Yakama	Pulmonary Tuberculosis
1929	18	F	Yakama	Tuberculosis
1929	2	M	Yakama	Tuberculosis
1929	18	M	Off Rez	Tuberculosis
1929	6	M	Yakama	Tuberculosis
1929	23	F	Yakama	Tuberculosis
1929	24	M	Yakama	Tuberculosis
1929	18	F	Yakama	Tuberculosis
1929	16	M	Off Rez	Tuberculosis
1930	30	F	Yakama	Tuberculosis
1930	4	F	Yakama	Tuberculosis
1930	32	F	Yakama	Tuberculosis
1930	1	M	Yakama	Tuberculosis
1930	29	M	Yakama	Tuberculosis
1930	54	F	Yakama	Tuberculosis
1930	32	M	Yakama	Tuberculosis
1930	57	M	Yakama	Tuberculosis
1930	45	M	Yakama	Tuberculosis
1930	30	F	Yakama	Pulmonary Tuberculosis
1930	30	F	Yakama	Tuberculosis
1930	29	M	Yakama	Pulmonary Tuberculosis
1930	36	F	Yakama	Pulmonary Tuberculosis
1930	45	F	Yakama	Tuberculosis
1930	54	F	Yakama	Pulmonary Tuberculosis
1930	57	M	Yakama	Tuberculosis
1930	35	F	Yakama	Pulmonary Tuberculosis
1930	32	F	Yakama	Pulmonary Tuberculosis
1930	5	F	Yakama	Pulmonary Tuberculosis
1930	47	M	Yakama	Tuberculosis

Year	Age	Gender	Place	Explanation
1930	22	F	Yakama	Pulmonary Tuberculosis
1930	2	M	Yakama	Tubercular Glands
1930	17	M	Yakama	Pulmonary Tuberculosis
1930	1	F	Yakama	Tuberculosis
1930	51	F	Yakama	Tuberculosis
1930	22	M	Yakama	Tuberculosis
1930	22	F	Yakama	—
1930	47	M	Yakama	Tuberculosis
1930	2	F	Yakama	Tuberculosis
1930	1	M	Yakama	Tuberculosis
1930	4	F	Yakama	Tuberculosis
1930	32	F	Yakama	Tuberculosis
1930	45	F	Yakama	Tuberculosis
1930	17	M	Yakama	Tuberculosis
1930	54	F	Yakama	Tuberculosis
1930	67	M	Yakama	Tuberculosis
1930	37	F	Yakama	Tuberculosis
1930	34	F	Yakama	Tuberculosis
1930	17	F	Yakama	Tuberculosis
1930	4	F	Off Rez	Tuberculosis
1930	16	M	Yakama	Tuberculosis
1931	51	F	Yakama	Tuberculosis
1931	64	F	Yakama	Tuberculosis
1931	16	M	Yakama	Tuberculosis
1931	16	M	Yakama	Tuberculosis
1931	24	M	Yakama	Tuberculosis
1931	18	F	Off Rez	Tuberculosis
1931	—	F	Off Rez	Tuberculosis
1931	55	M	Yakama	Tuberculosis
1931	17	F	Yakama	Tuberculosis
1931	17	F	Yakama	Tuberculosis
1931	35	M	Yakama	Tuberculosis
1931	15	M	Yakama	Tuberculosis
1931	41	F	Yakama	Tuberculosis
1931	24	M	Yakama	Pulmonary Tuberculosis
1931	0	F	Yakama	Tuberculosis
1931	16	M	Yakama	Tuberculosis
1931	55	M	Yakama	Tuberculosis
1931	25	M	Yakama	Pulmonary Tuberculosis
1931	36	F	Yakama	Tuberculosis

Year	Age	Gender	Place	Explanation
1931	17	F	Yakama	Pulmonary Tuberculosis
1931	15	M	Yakama	Pulmonary Tuberculosis
1931	35	M	Yakama	Pulmonary Tuberculosis
1931	16	M	Yakama	Pulmonary Tuberculosis
1931	17	F	Yakama	Pulmonary Tuberculosis
1931	18	F	Yakama	Pulmonary Tuberculosis
1931	16	M	Yakama	Pulmonary Tuberculosis
1932	25	M	Yakama	Tuberculosis
1932	49	M	Off Rez	Tuberculosis
1932	36	F	Yakama	Tuberculosis
1932	18	F	Off Rez	Tuberculosis
1932	19	M	Yakama	Tuberculosis
1932	17	M	Yakama	Tuberculosis
1932	11	F	Yakama	Tuberculosis
1932	70	M	Yakama	Tuberculosis
1932	7	F	Off Rez	Tuberculosis
1932	10	F	Yakama	Tuberculosis
1932	54	F	Yakama	Tuberculosis
1932	25	F	Yakama	Tuberculosis
1932	24	F	Yakama	Tuberculosis
1932	25	M	Yakama	Tuberculosis
1932	54	F	Yakama	Tuberculosis
1932	25	F	Yakama	Pulmonary Tuberculosis
1932	17	M	Yakama	Pulmonary Tuberculosis
1932	41	F	Yakama	Probably Tuberculosis
1932	10	F	Yakama	Probably Tuberculosis
1932	11	F	Yakama	Probably Tuberculosis
1932	19	M	Yakama	Intestinal Tuberculosis
1933	26	F	Yakama	Tuberculosis
1933	17	M	Yakama	Tuberculosis
1933	25	F	Off Rez	Tuberculosis
1933	58	F	Yakama	Tuberculosis
1933	—	M	Yakama	Tuberculosis
1933	23	M	Yakama	Tuberculosis
1933	75	M	Yakama	Tuberculosis
1933	29	F	Yakama	Tuberculosis
1933	75	M	Yakama	Tuberculosis
1933	25	F	Off Rez	Pulmonary Tuberculosis
1933	—	M	Yakama	Pulmonary Tuberculosis
1933	33	F	Yakama	Pulmonary Tuberculosis

Year	Age	Gender	Place	Explanation
1933	29	F	Off Rez	Pulmonary Tuberculosis
1933	23	M	Yakama	Pulmonary Tuberculosis
1933	17	M	Yakama	Pulmonary Tuberculosis
1933	58	F	Yakama	Pulmonary Tuberculosis
1933	27	F	Yakama	Pulmonary Tuberculosis
1934	8	F	Yakama	Tuberculosis
1934	24	F	Yakama	Tuberculosis
1934	26	M	Yakama	Tuberculosis
1934	27	M	Yakama	Tuberculosis
1934	41	F	Yakama	Tuberculosis
1934	21	M	Yakama	Tuberculosis
1934	50	F	Yakama	Tuberculosis
1934	27	M	Yakama	Tuberculosis
1934	18	M	Yakama	Tuberculosis
1934	30	M	Hospital	Tuberculosis
1934	9	M	Yakama	Tuberculosis
1934	19	F	Yakama	Tuberculosis
1934	46	F	Yakama	Pulmonary Tuberculosis
1934	19	F	Yakama	Pulmonary Tuberculosis
1934	9	M	Yakama	Chronic Pulmonary Tuberculosis
1934	27	M	Yakama	Pulmonary Tuberculosis
1934	8	F	Yakama	Pulmonary Tuberculosis
1934	21	M	Yakama	Pulmonary Tuberculosis
1934	24	F	Yakama	Pulmonary Tuberculosis
1934	41	F	Hospital	Pulmonary Tuberculosis
1934	18	M	Yakama	Pulmonary Tuberculosis
1934	27	M	Yakama	Pulmonary Tuberculosis
1934	26	M	Yakama	Pulmonary Tuberculosis
1935	35	F	Yakama	Tuberculosis
1935	27	F	Off Rez	Tuberculosis
1935	22	F	Yakama	Tuberculosis
1935	22	M	Yakama	Tuberculosis
1935	18	M	Yakama	Tuberculosis
1935	72	M	Yakama	Tuberculosis
1935	35	F	Yakama	Probably Tuberculosis
1935	72	M	Off Rez	Tuberculosis
1935	22	F	Yakama	Pulmonary Tuberculosis
1935	18	M	Yakama	Pulmonary Tuberculosis
1935	22	M	Yakama	Pulmonary Tuberculosis
1936	31	F	Off Rez	Tuberculosis

Year	Age	Gender	Place	Explanation
1936	57	M	Yakama	Tuberculosis
1936	27	M	Yakama	Tuberculosis
1936	27	F	Off Rez	Tuberculosis
1936	50	M	Yakama	Tuberculosis
1936	57	M	Yakama	Tuberculosis
1936	25	M	Yakama	Tuberculosis
1936	26	F	Yakama	Tuberculosis
1936	20	F	Yakama	Tuberculosis
1936	24	M	Yakama	Tuberculosis
1936	22	M	Yakama	Tuberculosis
1936	50	M	Yakama	Tuberculosis
1936	2	F	Off Rez	Tuberculosis
1937	35	M	Yakama	Tuberculosis
1937	20	F	Yakama	Tuberculosis
1937	31	M	Yakama	Tuberculosis
1937	10	F	Yakama	Tuberculosis
1937	2	F	Off Rez	Tuberculosis
1937	48	F	Off Rez	Tuberculosis
1937	37	F	Yakama	Tuberculosis
1937	22	F	Yakama	Tuberculosis
1937	12	M	Off Rez	Tuberculosis
1937	78	F	Off Rez	Tuberculosis
1937	15	F	Off Rez	Tuberculosis
1937	48	F	Yakama	Tuberculosis
1937	19	M	Yakama	Tuberculosis
1937	24	M	Yakama	Tuberculosis
1937	16	M	Off Rez	Tuberculosis
1937	69	M	Yakama	Tuberculosis
1937	10	F	Off Rez	Tuberculosis
1937	0	F	Yakama	Tuberculosis
1937	42	M	Yakama	Tuberculosis
1937	16	M	Off Rez	Tuberculosis
1937	48	F	Off Rez	Tuberculosis
1937	19	M	Yakama	Tuberculosis
1937	20	F	Yakama	Tuberculosis
1937	20	F	Yakama	Tuberculosis
1937	34	M	Yakama	Tuberculosis
1937	24	M	Yakama	Tuberculosis
1937	42	M	Yakama	Tuberculosis
1937	27	M	Off Rez	Tuberculosis

Year	Age	Gender	Place	Explanation
1937	35	M	Yakama	Tuberculosis
1937	34	M	Yakama	Tuberculosis
1937	20	F	Off Rez	Tuberculosis
1937	0	F	Yakama	Tuberculosis
1937	22	F	Yakama	Tuberculosis
1937	31	M	Hospital	Tuberculosis
1937	48	M	Yakama	Tuberculosis
1937	18	F	Yakama	Tuberculosis
1937	20	F	Yakama	Tuberculosis
1937	20	F	Yakama	Tuberculosis
1937	23	M	Yakama	Tuberculosis
1937	17	M	Yakama	Tuberculosis
1937	37	F	Yakama	Tuberculosis
1937	69	M	Yakama	Tuberculosis
1937	22	F	Yakama	Tuberculosis
1937	37	F	Yakama	Tuberculosis
1938	60	M	Off Rez	Tuberculosis
1938	5	M	Yakama	Tuberculosis
1938	77	F	Yakama	Tuberculosis
1938	52	M	Off Rez	Tuberculosis
1938	17	M	Yakama	Tuberculosis
1938	22	F	Yakama	Tuberculosis
1938	23	M	Yakama	Tuberculosis
1938	18	M	Yakama	Tuberculosis
1938	—	F	Yakama	Tuberculosis
1938	60	M	Off Rez	Tuberculosis
1938	22	F	Yakama	Tuberculosis
1938	20	F	Yakama	Tuberculosis
1938	18	M	Yakama	Tuberculosis
1938	5	M	Yakama	Tuberculosis
1938	22	F	Yakama	Tuberculosis
1939	76	M	Off Rez	Tuberculosis
1939	27	M	Off Rez	Tuberculosis
1939	31	F	Yakama	Tuberculosis
1939	36	M	Yakama	Tuberculosis
1939	19	M	Yakama	Tuberculosis
1939	80	F	Yakama	Tuberculosis
1939	23	M	Yakama	Tuberculosis
1939	20	M	Off Rez	Tuberculosis
1939	38	F	Yakama	Tuberculosis

Year	Age	Gender	Place	Explanation
1939	19	F	Off Rez	Tuberculosis
1939	14	F	Yakama	Tuberculosis
1939	29	M	Yakama	Tuberculosis
1939	27	M	Off Rez	Tuberculosis
1939	20	M	Off Rez	Tuberculosis
1939	80	F	Yakama	Tuberculosis
1939	19	M	Yakama	Tuberculosis
1939	38	F	Yakama	Tuberculosis
1939	4	F	Yakama	Tuberculosis
1939	31	F	Yakama	Tuberculosis
1939	14	F	Yakama	Tuberculosis
1939	76	M	Off Rez	Tuberculosis
1939	19	F	Off Rez	Tuberculosis
1939	55	M	Yakama	Tuberculosis
1939	36	M	Off Rez	Tuberculosis
1939	18	M	Yakama	Tuberculosis
1939	22	F	Yakama	Tuberculosis
1939	23	M	Yakama	Tuberculosis
1939	56	F	Yakama	Tuberculosis
1939	0	F	Yakama	Tuberculosis
1939	16	M	Yakama	Tuberculosis
1939	0	F	Yakama	Tuberculosis
1939	16	M	Yakama	Tuberculosis
1939	55	M	Yakama	Tuberculosis
1939	18	M	Yakama	Tuberculosis
1939	4	F	Yakama	Tuberculosis
1939	22	F	Yakama	Tuberculosis
1939	29	M	Off Rez	Tuberculosis
1939	56	F	Yakama	Tuberculosis
1940	26	M	Off Rez	Tuberculosis/Peritonitis
1940	71	F	Yakama	Tuberculosis
1940	0	M	Yakama	Tuberculosis
1940	18	F	Off Rez	Tuberculosis
1940	73	F	Off Rez	Tuberculosis
1940	62	F	Yakama	Tuberculosis/Diabetes
1940	14	F	Yakama	Tuberculosis
1940	0	F	Off Rez	Tuberculosis
1940	19	M	Yakama	Tuberculosis
1940	29	F	Off Rez	Tuberculosis
1940	62	F	Yakama	Tuberculosis

Year	Age	Gender	Place	Explanation
1940	0	M	Off Rez	Tuberculosis
1940	29	F	Off Rez	Tuberculosis
1940	39	F	Off Rez	Tuberculosis
1940	5	F	Off Rez	Tuberculosis
1940	19	M	Yakama	Tuberculosis
1940	18	F	Yakama	Tuberculosis
1940	17	M	Off Rez	Tuberculosis
1940	14	M	Yakama	Tuberculosis
1940	26	F	Off Rez	Tuberculosis
1940	0	M	Off Rez	Tuberculosis
1940	18	M	Off Rez	Tuberculosis
1940	17	M	Yakama	Tuberculosis
1940	18	F	Yakama	Tuberculosis
1940	39	F	Off Rez	Tuberculosis
1940	0	M	Yakama	Tuberculosis
1940	14	F	Yakama	Tuberculosis
1940	62	F	Yakama	Tuberculosis
1940	19	M	Yakama	Tuberculosis
1940	18	F	Yakama	Tuberculosis
1940	17	M	Yakama	Tuberculosis
1941	24	M	Off Rez	Tuberculosis
1941	28	M	Yakama	Tuberculosis
1941	18	F	Yakama	Tuberculosis
1941	16	M	Yakama	Tuberculosis
1941	23	M	Yakama	Tuberculosis
1941	55	F	Off Rez	Tuberculosis
1941	17	M	Yakama	Tuberculosis
1941	23	M	Yakama	Tuberculosis
1941	28	M	Yakama	Tuberculosis
1941	16	M	Yakama	Tuberculosis
1941	49	F	Yakama	Tuberculosis
1941	57	M	Off Rez	Tuberculosis
1941	25	F	Yakama	Tuberculosis
1941	19	M	Yakama	Tuberculosis
1941	49	F	Yakama	Tuberculosis
1941	25	F	Yakama	Tuberculosis
1941	25	F	Yakama	Tuberculosis
1941	18	F	Yakama	Tuberculosis
1941	57	M	Off Rez	Tuberculosis
1941	80	F	Off Rez	Tuberculosis

Year	Age	Gender	Place	Explanation
1941	19	M	Yakama	Tuberculosis
1941	15	M	Yakama	Tuberculosis
1941	23	M	Yakama	Tuberculosis
1941	9	M	Yakama	Tuberculosis/Nephritis
1942	39	F	Yakama	Tuberculosis
1942	22	M	Yakama	Tuberculosis
1942	7	F	Off Rez	Tuberculosis
1942	12	F	Yakama	Tuberculosis
1942	31	M	Yakama	Tuberculosis
1942	17	F	Yakama	Tuberculosis
1942	12	F	Yakama	Tuberculosis
1942	38	M	Yakama	Tuberculosis
1942	39	F	Yakama	Tuberculosis
1942	22	M	Yakama	Tuberculosis
1942	17	F	Yakama	Tuberculosis
1943	2	F	Yakama	Tuberculosis
1943	29	M	Off Rez	Tuberculosis
1943	56	F	Off Rez	Tuberculosis
1943	68	M	Off Rez	Tuberculosis
1943	13	F	Off Rez	Tuberculosis
1943	14	F	Yakama	Tuberculosis
1943	28	M	Yakama	Tuberculosis
1943	20	F	Yakama	Tuberculosis
1943	15	F	Off Rez	Tuberculosis
1943	26	F	Yakama	Tuberculosis
1943	28	F	Yakama	Tuberculosis
1943	22	F	Yakama	Tuberculosis
1943	28	F	Yakama	Tuberculosis
1943	22	M	Yakama	Tuberculosis
1943	48	M	Yakama	Tuberculosis
1943	48	M	Yakama	Tuberculosis
1943	57	F	Off Rez	Tuberculosis
1943	22	F	Yakama	Tuberculosis
1943	28	F	Yakama	Tuberculosis
1944	20	F	Yakama	Tuberculosis
1944	80	M	Off Rez	Tuberculosis
1944	81	F	Off Rez	Tuberculosis
1944	0	M	Yakama	Tuberculosis
1944	21	F	Yakama	Tuberculosis
1944	19	F	Off Rez	Tuberculosis

Year	Age	Gender	Place	Explanation
1944	21	F	Yakama	Tuberculosis
1944	18	F	Yakama	Tuberculosis
1944	61	F	Yakama	Tuberculosis
1944	18	F	Off Rez	Tuberculosis
1944	20	F	Yakama	Tuberculosis
1945	4	M	Off Rez	Tuberculosis
1945	41	F	Off Rez	Tuberculosis
1945	19	M	Off Rez	Tuberculosis
1945	55	F	Yakama	Tuberculosis
1945	22	F	Off Rez	Tuberculosis
1945	20	M	Off Rez	Tuberculosis
1945	76	F	Off Rez	Tuberculosis
1945	4	M	Yakama	Tuberculosis
1945	17	F	Off Rez	Tuberculosis
1945	1	M	Yakama	Tuberculosis
1946	13	F	Yakama	Tuberculosis
1946	1	F	Yakama	Tuberculosis
1946	36	F	Off Rez	Tuberculosis
1946	10	F	Yakama	Tuberculosis
1946	18	F	Off Rez	Tuberculosis
1946	17	M	Off Rez	Tuberculosis
1946	5	F	Off Rez	Tuberculosis
1946	17	M	Off Rez	Tuberculosis
1946	70	M	Off Rez	Tuberculosis
1947	38	F	Off Rez	Tuberculosis
1947	34	M	Off Rez	Tuberculosis
1947	73	F	Yakama	Tuberculosis
1947	34	F	Off Rez	Tuberculosis
1947	42	F	Yakama	Tuberculosis
1947	17	F	Off Rez	Tuberculosis
1947	26	F	Yakama	Tuberculosis
1947	52	M	Off Rez	Tuberculosis
1947	17	M	Off Rez	Tuberculosis
1948	25	M	Off Rez	Tuberculosis
1948	70	F	Yakama	Tuberculosis
1948	29	F	Off Rez	Tuberculosis
1948	78	F	Off Rez	Tuberculosis
1948	2	M	Off Rez	Tuberculosis
1948	66	M	Off Rez	Tuberculosis
1949	45	M	Yakama	Tuberculosis

Year	Age	Gender	Place	Explanation
1949	18	M	Off Rez	Tuberculosis
1949	4	F	Off Rez	Tuberculosis
1949	19	F	Off Rez	Tuberculosis
1949	24	M	Off Rez	Tuberculosis
1950	69	F	Yakama	Tuberculosis/Syphilis
1950	22	M	Off Rez	Tuberculosis
1950	75	F	Yakama	Tuberculosis
1951	26	M	Off Rez	Tuberculosis
1953	61	M	Yakama	Tuberculosis
1954	0	M	Yakama	Probably Pulmonary Tuberculosis
1957	17	M	Yakama	Pulmonary Tuberculosis
1959	60	M	Yakama	Signs of Pulmonary Tuberculosis
1960	82	F	Off Rez	Tuberculosis-Bronchopneumonia
1962	50	F	Hospital	Pulmonary Congestion/ Tuberculosis
1964	45	F	Hospital	Tuberculosis

Pneumonia

BETWEEN 1888 AND 1964, pneumonia flourished on the Yakama Indian Reservation. According to the clinical records of deaths on the reservation, pneumonia was the second largest killer, constituting approximately 26 percent of all deaths among the native people living on the reservation. However, many of the deaths recorded as caused by pneumonia among infants and children may well have been tuberculosis, disguised as pneumonia because of the lack of training by the recording person, including Indian agents and staff working for the Office of Indian Affairs. These individuals provided clinical descriptions of death based on information provided by family members, and recording agents provided the descriptions based on symptomatic descriptions, not autopsies, which would have offered medical explanations of death. Without the use of X-rays and autopsies, tuberculosis in infants and babies often appeared to be pneumonia. However, there is no way of knowing if pneumonia or tuberculosis caused the deaths of so many children historically on the reservation, but medical professionals specializing in respiratory diseases suggest that because tuberculosis was so prevalent on the reservation, infants and small children likely died of tuberculosis, not pneumonia.

Although poison gas may produce pneumonia, viral and bacterial infections caused the pneumonia on the Yakama Reservation. People died of lobar pneumonia and bronchopneumonia. Lobar pneumonia caused inflammation in one lobe of one lung that often spread to other lobes. Bronchopneumonia emerged in the bronchioles or bronchi (airways) of one or both lungs, spreading from infected areas to healthy tissues. Streptococcus pneumonia likely caused most of the bacterial pneumonia on the reservation, although other forms of the disease probably existed, including staphylococcus aureus and hemophilus influenzae. Regardless of the type, pneumonia generally caused inflammation of the lungs and other areas of the body, a dangerous condition wherever it occurred in the body. Individuals suffering from pneumonia often exhibited high fever, chills, coughs, sweats, and chest pain. People with pneumonia could also be short of breath, even in a reclined and resting position, and many coughed phlegm—sometimes bloody phlegm. In children, pneumonia sometimes created a blue tint to their lips and skin. The disease could cause delirium and a general disorientation. Pneumonia sometimes took the lives of people on the reservation already suffering from other conditions or ailments, including tuberculosis, cancer, bronchitis, influenza, or cancer. It struck the very young and the elderly. Death certificates from the Yakama Reservation generally indicated that a person simply died of pneumonia, but other times recorders provided secondary causes of death as "pneumonia and influenza," "pneumonia following measles," or "pneumonia and tuberculosis."

On the Yakama Reservation, infants and children suffered more deaths from pneumonia than any other age group, and the disease killed more males than females because it is more prevalent in boys—who are weaker biologically as infants—than girls during infancy and old age. Unlike tuberculosis, pneumonia deaths continued to be a factor among Yakama people throughout the 1940s and 1950s, in part because antibiotics could not control viral forms of pneumonia. Thus, in spite of advances in medicine during the mid-20th century and the development of public health, sanitation, housing, education, and health care, pneumonia remained a major killer into the 1960s.

Year	Age	Gender	Place	Explanation
1911	—	F	Yakama	Pneumonia
1915	58	F	Yakama	Pneumonia
1915	20	M	Yakama	Pneumonia
1915	60	M	Yakama	Pneumonia
1916	70	F	Yakama	Pneumonia
1916	7	F	Yakama	Pneumonia
1916	60	F	Yakama	Pneumonia
1916	4	M	Yakama	Pneumonia
1917	55	F	Yakama	Pneumonia
1917	2	F	Yakama	Pneumonia
1917	2	F	Yakama	Pneumonia
1917	1	F	Yakama	Pneumonia
1918	2	M	Yakama	Pneumonia
1918	1	M	Yakama	Pulmonary Pneumonia
1918	2	F	Yakama	Pulmonary Pneumonia
1918	6	M	Yakama	Pulmonary Pneumonia
1918	3	F	Yakama	Pulmonary Pneumonia
1918	6	M	Yakama	Pulmonary Pneumonia
1918	1	M	Yakama	Pulmonary Pneumonia
1918	1	F	Yakama	Pulmonary Pneumonia
1918	1	M	Yakama	Pulmonary Pneumonia
1918	1	M	Yakama	Pulmonary Pneumonia
1918	4	F	Yakama	Pulmonary Pneumonia
1918	15	F	Yakama	Pulmonary Pneumonia
1918	17	F	Yakama	Pulmonary Pneumonia
1918	5	M	Yakama	Pulmonary Pneumonia
1918	2	M	Yakama	Pulmonary Pneumonia
1919	53	M	Yakama	Pneumonia
1923	0	F	Yakama	Pneumonia
1924	0	F	Yakama	Pneumonia
1924	4	F	Yakama	Bronchopneumonia
1924	0	F	Yakama	Pneumonia and Measles
1924	4	M	Yakama	Pneumonia and Measles
1924	2	M	Yakama	Pneumonia
1924	1	M	Yakama	Pneumonia
1924	3	F	Yakama	Pneumonia
1924	69	M	Yakama	Pneumonia
1924	1	M	Yakama	Pneumonia
1924	1	F	Yakama	Pneumonia
1924	9	M	Yakama	Pneumonia

Year	Age	Gender	Place	Explanation
1924	0	F	Yakama	Pneumonia
1925	18	F	Yakama	Pneumonia
1925	58	F	Yakama	Pneumonia
1925	9	F	Yakama	Pneumonia
1925	8	F	Yakama	Pneumonia
1925	0	M	Yakama	Pneumonia
1925	0	F	Yakama	Pneumonia
1925	0	F	Yakama	Pneumonia
1925	0	M	Yakama	Pneumonia
1925	1	M	Yakama	Pneumonia
1925	0	F	Yakama	Pneumonia
1925	1	F	Yakama	Pneumonia
1925	0	M	Yakama	Pneumonia
1925	1	F	Yakama	Pneumonia
1925	58	F	Yakama	Pneumonia
1925	1	M	Yakama	Pneumonia
1925	4	M	Yakama	Pneumonia
1925	5	F	Yakama	Bronchopneumonia
1925	0	M	Yakama	Acute Pneumonia
1925	51	F	Yakama	Pneumonia
1925	51	F	Off Rez	Bronchopneumonia
1925	1	F	Yakama	Pneumonia
1925	4	M	Yakama	Pneumonia
1925	2	F	Yakama	Pneumonia
1926	2	F	Yakama	Pneumonia
1926	1	F	Yakama	Pneumonia
1926	1	F	Yakama	Pneumonia
1926	2	F	Yakama	Pneumonia
1926	1	M	Yakama	Pneumonia
1926	28	M	Yakama	Pneumonia
1926	1	M	Yakama	Pneumonia
1926	0	F	Yakama	Pneumonia
1926	2	M	Yakama	Lobar Pneumonia
1926	2	M	Yakama	Pneumonia
1926	1	F	Yakama	Pneumonia
1926	4	F	Yakama	Bronchopneumonia
1926	38	F	Yakama	Pneumonia
1926	1	M	Yakama	Pneumonia
1926	0	F	Yakama	Pneumonia
1926	0	F	Yakama	Pneumonia

Year	Age	Gender	Place	Explanation
1926	3	F	Yakama	Bronchopneumonia
1926	1	F	Yakama	Pneumonia
1926	34	F	Yakama	Pneumonia
1926	0	M	Yakama	Pneumonia
1926	1	M	Yakama	Pneumonia
1926	2	M	Yakama	Pneumonia
1926	0	M	Yakama	Pneumonia
1926	0	M	Yakama	Pneumonia
1926	0	M	Yakama	Pneumonia
1926	0	M	Yakama	Pneumonia
1926	25	M	Yakama	Pneumonia
1926	32	F	Yakama	Pneumonia
1927	28	F	Off Rez	Pneumonia
1927	2	F	Yakama	Pneumonia
1927	85	M	Yakama	Acute Pneumonia
1927	2	F	Yakama	Pneumonia
1927	1	F	Yakama	Lobar Pneumonia
1927	69	F	Yakama	Pneumonia
1928	49	F	Yakama	Lobar Pneumonia
1928	1	M	Yakama	Pneumonia
1928	65	M	Yakama	Pneumonia
1928	0	F	Yakama	Pneumonia
1928	60	M	Yakama	Pneumonia
1928	49	F	Yakama	Lobar Pneumonia
1928	0	M	Yakama	Pneumonia
1928	0	M	Yakama	Pneumonia
1928	27	F	Yakama	Pneumonia
1928	0	M	Yakama	Pneumonia
1928	4	M	Yakama	Pneumonia
1928	85	F	Yakama	Pneumonia
1928	0	F	Yakama	Pneumonia
1928	0	F	Yakama	Pneumonia
1928	57	F	Yakama	Pneumonia
1928	3	F	Yakama	Acute Bronchopneumonia
1928	43	M	Yakama	Pneumonia and Tuberculosis
1928	44	M	Yakama	—
1928	70	F	Yakama	—
1928	24	M	Yakama	—
1928	3	M	Yakama	—
1928	6	M	Yakama	—

Year	Age	Gender	Place	Explanation
1928	1	M	Yakama	—
1928	1	F	Yakama	—
1928	57	F	Yakama	—
1928	83	F	Off Rez	Senility and Pneumonia
1928	1	F	Off Rez	Pneumonia
1928	68	F	Off Rez	Pneumonia
1928	44	M	Off Rez	Pneumonia
1928	1	F	Off Rez	Pneumonia
1928	78	F	Off Rez	Pneumonia and Influenza
1928	0	M	Off Rez	Pneumonia
1928	20	F	Off Rez	Pneumonia
1929	3	M	Yakama	—
1929	1	M	Yakama	—
1929	76	F	Off Rez	—
1929	64	M	Yakama	—
1929	6	M	Yakama	Bronchopneumonia
1929	48	M	Yakama	Bronchopneumonia
1929	0	F	Yakama	Pneumonia
1929	0	M	Yakama	Bronchopneumonia
1929	64	M	Yakama	Lobar Pneumonia
1929	3	M	Yakama	Bronchopneumonia
1929	0	M	Yakama	Bronchopneumonia
1929	44	M	Yakama	Pneumonia
1929	0	M	Yakama	Acute Bronchopneumonia
1929	0	F	Yakama	Bronchopneumonia
1929	0	M	Yakama	Bronchopneumonia
1929	21	M	Off Rez	Pneumonia
1929	0	F	Off Rez	Pneumonia
1929	2	M	Yakama	Bronchopneumonia
1930	2	F	Yakama	Bronchopneumonia
1930	0	M	Yakama	Bronchopneumonia
1930	2	F	Yakama	Bronchopneumonia
1930	2	M	Yakama	Bronchopneumonia
1930	2	M	Yakama	Lobar Pneumonia
1930	0	M	Yakama	Bronchopneumonia
1930	2	M	Yakama	Bronchopneumonia
1930	0	F	Yakama	Bronchopneumonia
1930	59	M	Yakama	Supposed Pneumonia
1930	1	M	Yakama	Pneumonia
1930	1	M	Yakama	Pneumonia

Year	Age	Gender	Place	Explanation
1930	4	F	Yakama	Said to Be Pneumonia
1930	2	M	Yakama	Pneumonia
1930	3	F	Yakama	Pneumonia
1930	0	F	Yakama	Pneumonia
1930	0	M	Yakama	Pneumonia
1930	0	F	Yakama	Pneumonia
1930	0	M	Yakama	Pneumonia
1930	59	M	Yakama	Pneumonia
1930	0	F	Yakama	Pneumonia
1930	86	F	Yakama	Pneumonia
1930	2	M	Yakama	Pneumonia
1930	0	M	Yakama	Pneumonia
1930	82	M	Off Rez	Pneumonia
1931	2	M	Yakama	Pneumonia
1931	3	M	Yakama	Pneumonia
1931	37	F	Yakama	Pneumonia
1931	2	M	Yakama	Pneumonia
1931	1	M	Yakama	Pneumonia
1931	0	M	Yakama	Bronchopneumonia
1931	2	F	Yakama	Pneumonia
1931	0	F	Yakama	Pneumonia
1931	1	M	Yakama	Pneumonia
1931	1	F	Yakama	Pneumonia
1931	1	F	Off Rez	Pneumonia
1931	70	F	Off Rez	Pneumonia
1931	0	M	Yakama	Pneumonia
1931	36	F	Off Rez	Pneumonia
1931	2	M	Yakama	Pneumonia
1931	0	M	Yakama	Pneumonia
1931	1	M	Yakama	Pneumonia
1931	1	M	Yakama	Pneumonia
1931	0	0	Yakama	Pneumonia
1931	0	M	Yakama	Said to Be Pneumonia
1931	3	F	Yakama	Said to Be Pneumonia
1931	3	M	Yakama	Said to Be Pneumonia
1931	0	M	Yakama	Pneumonia
1931	0	M	Yakama	Not Bronchopneumonia
1931	2	M	Yakama	Bronchopneumonia
1931	1	M	Yakama	Bronchopneumonia
1931	1	M	Yakama	Bronchopneumonia

Year	Age	Gender	Place	Explanation
1931	7	M	Yakama	Bronchopneumonia
1931	1	M	Yakama	Acute Bronchopneumonia
1932	0	F	Yakama	Pneumonia
1932	0	M	Yakama	Pneumonia
1932	0	M	Yakama	Pneumonia
1932	0	M	Yakama	Pneumonia
1932	0	F	Yakama	Pneumonia
1932	70	M	Yakama	Pneumonia
1932	0	M	Yakama	Pneumonia
1932	0	M	Yakama	Pneumonia
1932	0	—	Yakama	Probably Pneumonia
1932	0	M	Yakama	Probably Pneumonia
1932	0	M	Yakama	Bronchopneumonia
1932	0	M	Yakama	Probably Pneumonia
1932	0	M	Yakama	Probably Pneumonia
1932	70	M	Yakama	Lobar Pneumonia
1933	26	F	Yakama	Pneumonia
1933	27	F	Yakama	Pneumonia
1934	5	F	Yakama	Pneumonia
1934	1	F	Yakama	Pneumonia
1934	50	M	Yakama	Pneumonia
1934	61	M	Yakama	Pneumonia
1934	24	M	Yakama	Pneumonia
1934	3	M	Yakama	Pneumonia
1934	7	F	Yakama	Pneumonia
1934	61	M	Yakama	Pneumonia
1934	7	F	Yakama	Bronchopneumonia
1934	1	F	Yakama	Bronchopneumonia
1934	24	M	Yakama	Lobar Pneumonia
1935	3	F	Yakama	Pneumonia
1935	0	M	Off Rez	Pneumonia
1935	42	M	Yakama	Pneumonia
1935	80	M	Yakama	Pneumonia
1935	0	M	Yakama	Pneumonia
1935	68	M	Yakama	Pneumonia/Tuberculosis
1935	0	M	Yakama	Pneumonia
1935	3	F	Yakama	Bronchopneumonia
1935	68	M	Yakama	Lobar Pneumonia
1935	0	M	Yakama	Bronchopneumonia
1935	80	M	Off Rez	Bronchopneumonia

Year	Age	Gender	Place	Explanation
1935	42	—	Hospital	Lobar Pneumonia
1936	6	F	Yakama	Pneumonia
1936	10	M	Off Rez	Pneumonia
1936	50	M	Yakama	Pneumonia
1936	0	M	Yakama	Pneumonia
1936	73	F	Hospital	Pneumonia
1936	1	M	Yakama	Pneumonia
1936	28	F	Yakama	Pneumonia
1936	29	F	Yakama	Pneumonia
1936	50	M	Yakama	Pneumonia
1936	22	M	Yakama	Pneumonia
1936	50	M	Yakama	Pneumonia
1936	22	M	Yakama	Pneumonia
1936	28	F	Yakama	Pneumonia
1936	6	F	Yakama	Pneumonia
1936	1	F	Yakama	Pneumonia
1936	50	M	Yakama	Pneumonia
1936	1	M	Yakama	Pneumonia
1936	59	M	Yakama	Pneumonia
1936	22	M	Yakama	Pneumonia
1936	0	M	Yakama	Pneumonia
1937	72	M	Yakama	Pneumonia
1937	41	F	Yakama	Pneumonia
1937	78	M	Yakama	Pneumonia
1937	0	M	Yakama	Pneumonia/Enteritis
1937	88	M	Yakama	Pneumonia
1937	42	M	Yakama	Pneumonia
1937	23	M	Yakama	Pneumonia
1937	75	M	Yakama	Pneumonia
1937	75	M	Yakama	Pneumonia
1937	3	M	Yakama	Pneumonia
1937	42	M	Yakama	Pneumonia
1937	0	M	Yakama	Pneumonia
1937	78	M	Yakama	Pneumonia
1937	72	M	Yakama	Pneumonia
1937	75	M	Yakama	Pneumonia
1937	3	M	Yakama	Pneumonia
1937	57	F	Yakama	Pneumonia
1937	88	M	Yakama	Pneumonia
1937	41	F	Off Rez	Pneumonia

Year	Age	Gender	Place	Explanation
1937	0	M	Yakama	Pneumonia
1937	47	F	Yakama	Pneumonia
1937	74	F	Yakama	Pneumonia
1938	1	M	Yakama	Pneumonia
1938	87	F	Off Rez	Pneumonia
1938	0	M	Yakama	Pneumonia
1938	0	M	Yakama	Pneumonia
1938	74	F	Yakama	Pneumonia
1938	0	F	Yakama	Pneumonia/Whooping Cough
1938	87	F	Off Rez	Pneumonia
1938	1	M	Yakama	Pneumonia
1938	47	F	Yakama	Pneumonia/Tuberculosis/Heart Disease
1938	0	M	Yakama	Pneumonia
1939	0	F	Hospital	Pneumonia
1939	76	F	Off Rez	Pneumonia
1939	82	M	Off Rez	Pneumonia
1939	69	M	Off Rez	Pneumonia
1939	1	M	Yakama	Pneumonia
1939	0	M	Yakama	Enterocolitis/Pneumonia
1939	0	M	Yakama	Enterocolitis/Pneumonia
1939	36	F	Yakama	Pneumonia
1939	55	M	Yakama	Pneumonia
1939	82	M	Off Rez	Pneumonia
1939	1	M	Yakama	Pneumonia
1939	36	F	Yakama	Pneumonia
1939	55	M	Yakama	Pneumonia
1939	76	F	Off Rez	Pneumonia/Heart Disease
1939	70	M	Yakama	Pneumonia
1939	0	M	Yakama	Enterocolitis/Pneumonia
1939	82	F	Off Rez	Pneumonia
1939	82	F	Off Rez	Pneumonia
1939	82	F	Off Rez	Pneumonia
1939	56	M	Yakama	Pneumonia
1940	3	F	Off Rez	Pneumonia
1940	42	F	Off Rez	Pneumonia
1940	65	F	Off Rez	Pneumonia
1940	46	M	Yakama	Pneumonia
1940	0	M	Yakama	Pneumonia
1940	1	F	Yakama	Pneumonia

Year	Age	Gender	Place	Explanation
1940	4	M	Yakama	Pneumonia
1940	48	F	Yakama	Pneumonia
1940	0	F	Yakama	Pneumonia
1940	0	F	Off Rez	Pneumonia
1940	42	F	Off Rez	Pneumonia
1940	4	M	Yakama	Pneumonia
1940	46	M	Yakama	Pneumonia
1940	3	F	Off Rez	Pneumonia
1940	0	M	Off Rez	Pneumonia/Measles
1940	65	F	Off Rez	Pneumonia/Syphilis
1940	48	F	Yakama	Pneumonia
1940	95	M	Yakama	Pneumonia
1940	0	F	Yakama	Pneumonia
1940	59	F	Yakama	Pneumonia
1940	—	F	Yakama	Pneumonia
1940	42	F	Off Rez	Pneumonia
1940	44	M	Yakama	Pneumonia
1941	0	M	Yakama	Pneumonia
1941	0	M	Yakama	Pneumonia
1941	0	M	Yakama	Pneumonia/Gastroenteritis
1941	77	F	Yakama	Pneumonia
1941	0	F	Yakama	Pneumonia
1941	73	M	Yakama	Pneumonia
1941	0	M	Yakama	Pneumonia/Gastroenteritis
1941	77	F	Off Rez	Pneumonia
1941	0	M	Yakama	Pneumonia
1941	0	M	Off Rez	Pneumonia
1941	0	M	Yakama	Pneumonia/Gastroenteritis
1942	56	M	Off Rez	Pneumonia
1942	68	M	Off Rez	Pneumonia
1942	18	F	Yakama	Pneumonia/Tuberculosis
1942	0	M	Off Rez	Pneumonia
1942	0	F	Off Rez	Pneumonia
1942	47	F	Yakama	Pneumonia/Syphilis
1942	68	F	Yakama	Pneumonia
1942	0	F	Yakama	Pneumonia
1942	58	M	Yakama	Pneumonia
1942	68	F	Yakama	Pneumonia
1942	9	F	Off Rez	Pneumonia
1942	11	F	Off Rez	Pneumonia/Tuberculosis

Year	Age	Gender	Place	Explanation
1942	0	F	Yakama	Pneumonia
1942	0	F	Off Rez	Pneumonia
1942	18	F	Yakama	Pneumonia/Tuberculosis
1943	0	M	Yakama	Pneumonia [Probably Crib Death]
1943	0	F	Yakama	Pneumonia/Dysentery
1943	0	F	Off Rez	Pneumonia
1943	26	F	Off Rez	Pneumonia
1943	1	F	Off Rez	Pneumonia/Whooping Cough
1943	26	M	Off Rez	Pneumonia
1943	0	F	Yakama	Pneumonia
1943	0	M	Off Rez	Pneumonia
1943	0	F	Yakama	Pneumonia
1943	1	F	Off Rez	Pneumonia
1944	1	M	Yakama	Pneumonia
1944	1	F	Off Rez	Pneumonia
1944	1	M	Yakama	Pneumonia
1944	0	F	Yakama	Pneumonia
1944	0	M	Off Rez	Pneumonia
1944	2	M	Yakama	Pneumonia
1944	1	M	Off Rez	Pneumonia
1944	0	M	Off Rez	Pneumonia
1944	—	F	Yakama	Pneumonia
1944	0	M	Yakama	Pneumonia
1944	69	M	Off Rez	Pneumonia
1944	1	M	Yakama	Pneumonia
1944	0	F	Yakama	Pneumonia
1944	0	M	Yakama	Pneumonia
1944	1	M	Yakama	Pneumonia
1944	0	M	Yakama	Pneumonia
1944	0	M	Yakama	Pneumonia
1944	80	F	Yakama	Pneumonia
1944	0	M	Yakama	Pneumonia
1945	1	M	Yakama	Pneumonia/Dysentery
1945	0	M	Yakama	Pneumonia
1945	0	F	Off Rez	Pneumonia
1945	0	F	Yakama	Pneumonia
1945	57	F	Yakama	Pneumonia
1945	0	M	Yakama	Pneumonia
1945	98	F	Off Rez	Pneumonia/Gangrene
1945	3	F	Off Rez	Pneumonia/Croup

Year	Age	Gender	Place	Explanation
1945	54	M	Off Rez	Pneumonia
1945	76	F	Yakama	Pneumonia
1945	58	M	Off Rez	Pneumonia/Cerebral Hemorrhage
1945	69	F	Yakama	Pneumonia
1945	1	F	Yakama	Pneumonia
1945	0	M	Yakama	Pneumonia
1945	0	M	Off Rez	Pneumonia
1946	3	F	Off Rez	Pneumonia
1946	0	F	Off Rez	Pneumonia
1946	0	F	Yakama	Pneumonia
1946	58	F	Yakama	Pneumonia
1946	0	M	Off Rez	Pneumonia
1946	80	F	Yakama	Pneumonia
1946	0	M	Yakama	Pneumonia
1946	0	M	Off Rez	Pneumonia
1946	0	F	Yakama	Pneumonia/Breech Childbirth
1946	0	F	Yakama	Pneumonia
1947	0	M	Off Rez	Pneumonia
1947	0	M	Yakama	Pneumonia
1947	50	M	Yakama	Pneumonia
1947	0	M	Yakama	Pneumonia
1947	70	M	Off Rez	Pneumonia
1948	3	M	Yakama	Pneumonia
1948	70	M	Off Rez	Pneumonia
1948	46	F	Off Rez	Pneumonia/Heart Disease
1949	0	M	Yakama	Pneumonia
1949	0	M	Yakama	Pneumonia
1949	2	M	Yakama	Pneumonia
1949	0	M	Yakama	Pneumonia
1949	85	F	Off Rez	Pneumonia
1949	0	M	Yakama	Pneumonia
1949	0	M	Off Rez	Pneumonia
1949	54	M	Off Rez	Pneumonia
1950	0	F	Yakama	Pneumonia
1950	0	F	Yakama	Pneumonia
1950	0	M	Yakama	Pneumonia
1950	71	F	Yakama	Pneumonia
1950	0	F	Yakama	Pneumonia
1951	0	M	Off Rez	Pneumonia
1951	76	M	Yakama	Pneumonia

Year	Age	Gender	Place	Explanation
1951	0	M	Yakama	Pneumonia/Pituitary Disorder
1951	55	F	Yakama	Pneumonia
1952	90	F	Yakama	Pneumonia
1952	1	F	Yakama	Pneumonia
1952	0	F	Yakama	Pneumonia
1952	0	M	Yakama	Pneumonia
1952	0	M	Yakama	Pneumonia/Malnutrition
1952	0	M	Yakama	Pneumonia
1952	0	F	Yakama	Pleurisy/Pneumonia
1952	0	M	Yakama	Pneumonia
1952	0	M	Yakama	Pneumonia Enteritis
1952	54	M	Off Rez	Pneumonia
1952	72	M	Yakama	Pneumonia
1953	0	M	Yakama	Pneumonia/Improper Care
1953	1	F	Yakama	Pneumonia/Measles
1953	73	M	Off Rez	Uremia/Prostrate Hypertrophy
1953	0	M	Yakama	Pneumonia
1953	0	M	Yakama	Pneumonia
1953	0	F	Yakama	Pneumonia
1953	0	M	Yakama	Pneumonia
1953	1	F	Yakama	Pneumonia/Heart Disease
1953	0	M	Off Rez	Pneumonia/Heart Disease
1953	0	M	Yakama	Pneumonia/Malnutrition
1954	0	M	Yakama	Probably Bronchopneumonia
1954	42	M	Yakama	Pneumonia/Nephritis
1954	0	M	Yakama	Signs of Pneumonia
1954	76	F	Yakama	Bronchopneumonia
1954	68	F	Off Rez	Pneumonia
1954	0	F	Off Rez	Pneumonia
1954	0	M	Yakama	Possibly Bronchopneumonia
1954	2	F	Off Rez	Pneumonia
1955	60	M	Yakama	Probably Pneumonia
1955	0	M	Yakama	Signs of Pneumonia
1955	0	M	Off Rez	Pneumonia
1955	0	M	Off Rez	Bronchopneumonia
1955	0	M	Yakama	Signs of Bronchopneumonia
1955	0	M	Off Rez	Bilateral Bronchopneumonia
1955	0	M	Yakama	Pneumonia
1955	4	F	Yakama	Pneumonia
1955	0	M	Yakama	Possibly Bronchopneumonia

Year	Age	Gender	Place	Explanation
1955	0	F	Yakama	Probably Bronchopneumonia
1956	48	M	Off Rez	Pneumonia/Cerebral Hemorrhage
1956	77	F	Yakama	Possibly Bronchopneumonia
1956	0	F	Off Rez	Bronchopneumonia
1956	0	M	Yakama	Signs of Pneumonia
1956	71	M	Off Rez	Pneumonia/Myocarditis/Nephritis
1956	0	M	Yakama	Acute Intestinal Pneumonia
1956	0	F	Off Rez	Pneumonia
1956	0	F	Off Rez	Lobar Pneumonia
1956	0	M	Yakama	Probably Bronchopneumonia
1956	0	F	Off Rez	Pneumonia
1956	0	F	Off Rez	Pneumonia Aspiration
1957	0	F	Off Rez	Bronchopneumonia
1957	40	F	Off Rez	Bilateral Pneumonia/Alcohol Problems
1957	4	M	Yakama	Pneumonia
1957	0	M	Yakama	Signs of Pneumonia
1957	0	F	Off Rez	Pneumonia/Malnutrition
1957	54	M	Off Rez	Pneumonia/Cardiac Failure
1957	0	F	Off Rez	Possible Bronchopneumonia
1957	0	F	Off Rez	Pneumonitis
1957	35	F	Yakama	Virus Pneumonia
1957	0	F	Off Rez	Pneumonia/Measles
1957	0	M	Off Rez	Virus Pneumonia/Bronchitis
1958	0	M	Yakama	Signs of Pneumonia
1958	2	F	Yakama	Pneumonia
1958	57	M	Off Rez	Acute Pneumonia/Tuberculosis
1958	0	M	Off Rez	Pneumonia
1958	0	F	Off Rez	Pneumonia
1958	0	F	Off Rez	Bronchopneumonia
1958	80	M	Off Rez	Bronchopneumonia
1958	0	F	Off Rez	Bilateral Bronchopneumonia
1958	0	F	Off Rez	Bronchopneumonia
1958	0	M	Off Rez	Signs of Bronchopneumonia
1959	0	M	Yakama	Bronchopneumonia
1959	0	M	Yakama	Signs of Bronchopneumonia
1959	6	M	Yakama	Bronchopneumonia
1959	88	F	Off Rez	Pneumonitis
1960	0	M	Yakama	Pneumonia
1960	0	M	Hospital	Pneumonia/Malnutrition

Year	Age	Gender	Place	Explanation
1960	0	F	Off Rez	Pneumonia/Gastroenteritis
1960	0	M	Hospital	Signs of Pneumonia
1960	7	F	Off Rez	Pneumonia/Cardiac Failure
1960	0	M	Hospital	Pneumonia
1960	56	M	Off Rez	Pneumonia/Arteriosclerosis
1961	91	M	Hospital	Bronchopneumonia/Heart Failure
1961	89	M	Off Rez	Heart Failure/Bronchopneumonia
1961	24	M	Hospital	Bronchopneumonia
1961	0	M	Off Rez	Signs of Bronchopneumonia
1961	0	M	Off Rez	Terminal Pneumonia
1961	73	M	Hospital	Probably Pneumonia
1961	0	M	Hospital	Bronchopneumonia
1961	0	M	Off Rez	Pneumonia/Enteritis
1961	0	M	Hospital	Signs of Bronchopneumonia
1962	91	F	Off Rez	Respiratory Failure/ Bronchopneumonia
1962	0	M	Off Rez	Bronchopneumonia/Malnutrition
1962	0	F	Hospital	Bronchopneumonia
1962	63	M	Off Rez	Pneumonia
1962	0	M	Hospital	Signs of Bronchopneumonia
1962	0	M	Hospital	Signs of Bronchopneumonia
1962	0	M	Off Rez	Bronchopneumonia
1962	0	F	Hospital	Possibly Bronchopneumonia
1962	87	F	Off Rez	Bronchopneumonia
1962	66	F	Off Rez	Bronchopneumonia
1962	0	F	Hospital	Possibly Bronchopneumonia
1962	86	F	Hospital	Bronchopneumonia
1962	0	F	Hospital	Possibly Bronchopneumonia
1962	87	F	Off Rez	Bronchopneumonia
1962	66	F	Off Rez	Bronchopneumonia
1963	62	M	Hospital	Bronchopneumonia
1963	0	M	Off Rez	Pneumonia/Dehydration/Diarrhea
1963	69	M	Hospital	Bronchopneumonia/Exposure
1963	4	F	Off Rez	Bronchopneumonia
1963	65	F	Off Rez	Bronchopneumonia
1963	0	F	Hospital	Pneumonitis
1963	0	M	Hospital	Signs of Bronchopneumonia
1963	0	M	Off Rez	Bronchopneumonia
1963	66	M	Hospital	Bronchopneumonia
1963	55	M	Off Rez	Lobar Pneumonia

Year	Age	Gender	Place	Explanation
1963	44	F	Off Rez	Pneumonia
1963	0	F	Hospital	Signs of Bronchopneumonia
1963	0	M	Off Rez	Intestinal Pneumonitis
1963	0	M	Off Rez	Pneumonia
1963	99	M	Hospital	Bronchopneumonia/Senility
1963	76	M	Off Rez	Bronchopneumonia/Senility
1964	75	M	Off Rez	Bilateral Bronchopneumonia
1964	0	M	Hospital	Probably Bronchopneumonia
1964	26	M	Off Rez	Bronchopneumonia
1964	99	F	Off Rez	Pneumonia/CVA/Arteriosclerosis
1964	0	M	Hospital	Probably Pneumonitis
1964	99	M	Hospital	Bronchopneumonia/Rheumatic Fever

Heart Disease

DURING THE ERA FROM 1888 TO 1964, heart disease was the third leading killer of American Indian people living on the Yakama Indian Reservation. Heart disease included congenital heart disease, heart failure, heart attacks, and other maladies affecting the heart. About 15 percent of all Indians that died during the period died of heart disease. Most likely, heart disease resulted in part from the stress created by the forced removal of Indian people to the reservation, war that raged between the United States and many Plateau Indian tribes in the 1850s, and the destruction of food resources during the late 19th and 20th centuries. The loss of foods affected Indian people in two major ways. For one, the bodies of Indian people had evolved biologically in such a way as to need and use roots, berries, venison, salmon, and other natural foods. Plateau Indians knew how to grow corn and raise other crops, but they derived most of their foods from their rich environment. As a result of the Plateau Indian War and forced removal to the reservations, Indians living on the Yakama Reservation lost their native foods. This development occurred over time, but the net result of the loss of native foods and other resources placed their bodies in jeopardy. Diet is a significant factor today in the development of heart disease, and although no clinical tests can be made on the bodies of people that lived in the past, we know that diet is and was a major factor contributing to heart disease.

Furthermore, the issue of native foods had another influence on heart disease. The loss of native foods had a tremendous psychological and spiritual impact on Indian people. In accordance with *tamanwit*, or native law, Indians were supposed to have a close relationship with all their foods. In fact, they were supposed to conduct yearly ceremonies to thank the creative force for the foods and thank the foods themselves through First Salmon Ceremonies, Root Ceremonies, and other thanksgiving ceremonies to perpetuate their lives and those of the species that the people consumed. This provided a balance that was important to the health of people, plants, and animals. The spiritual importance of this balance cannot be overstated because the Indian world on the plateau had always been closely associated with the natural environment. When the United States pushed the people from their traditional lands where they lived, fished, hunted, and gathered, the government contributed greatly to the ill health of the people in general and to heart diseases in particular. The mental and physical health of Yakama people declined dramatically as a result of the reservation system, creating conditions conducive to heart ailments of all kinds.

Weakened hearts resulted from malnutrition and stress of pregnant mothers on the Yakama Indian Reservation, who gave birth to babies with birth defects and heart diseases. However, agents recorded heart disease as the cause of death of only a few infants and small children during the period under investigation. Instead, most deaths from heart disease occurred among those individuals 55 years of age and older. According to documents found in the National Archives, nearly 70 percent of all those who died of heart disease on the Yakama Reservation from 1888 to 1964 were 55 years of age or older. Tobacco use was not a major factor causing heart disease on the reservation, at least not until after World War II, when traders brought larger quantities of tobacco onto the reservation. Furthermore, after World War II, Yakamas became influenced by mass marketing, and some former soldiers and sailors returned home with a habit they had cultivated in the armed forces when the United States government commonly gave military personnel cigarettes as part of their rations. Deaths resulting from heart disease increased during the course of the 20th century. Between 1911, when the agency recorded its first death from heart disease of a male nearly 100 years old, and 1949, a total of 198 people died of heart disease. Between 1950 and 1964 alone, 126 Yakama people died of heart disease. While deaths due to tuberculosis and most infectious diseases declined during the 1950s, deaths resulting from heart disease grew and became a major killer of the people. Heart disease remained a significant cause of death among Indian people of the Yakama Reservation during the late 20th and early 21st centuries.

Year	Age	Gender	Place	Explanation
1911	99	M	Yakama	Arteriosclerosis
1915	—	—	Yakama	Heart Failure
1915	80	M	Yakama	Heart Failure
1916	65	M	Yakama	Heart Failure
1917	79	M	Yakama	Heart Failure
1918	50	M	Yakama	Heart Failure
1920	47	M	Yakama	Angina Pectoris
1924	0	F	Yakama	Weak Heart
1924	63	M	Yakama	Chronic Myocarditis
1925	61	F	Yakama	Organic Heart Disease
1925	60	M	Yakama	Heart Trouble
1925	60	M	Yakama	Heart Trouble
1926	76	M	Yakama	Myocarditis
1926	90	M	Yakama	Hepatic Cirrhosis
1926	80	F	Yakama	Myocarditis
1926	66	F	Yakama	Myocarditis
1927	40	M	Yakama	Myocarditis
1927	82	F	Yakama	Myocarditis
1927	69	F	Yakama	Myocarditis
1927	82	F	Yakama	Chronic Myocarditis
1928	35	F	Yakama	Myocarditis
1928	35	F	Yakama	—
1928	99	F	Off Rez	Heart Disease
1928	7	F	Off Rez	Heart Disease
1928	89	F	Off Rez	Cardiac Asthma and Injuries
1928	35	F	Yakama	Heart Disease
1929	23	M	Yakama	Phthisis Pulmonalis
1929	69	M	Yakama	Pulmonary Congestion
1929	85	M	Yakama	Chronic Mitral Valve Lesion
1929	84	M	Yakama	Chronic Mitral Valve Lesion
1929	57	F	Yakama	Myocarditis
1929	79	M	Yakama	Myocarditis
1929	24	M	Off Rez	Phthisis Pulmonalis
1929	79	M	Yakama	Heart Disease
1929	57	F	Off Rez	Heart Disease
1930	75	M	Yakama	Organic Heart Trouble
1930	63	F	Yakama	Chronic Valvular Heart Disease
1930	65	M	Yakama	Organic Heart Trouble
1930	63	F	Yakama	Chronic Valvular Heart Disease
1930	70	M	Yakama	Heart Trouble

Year	Age	Gender	Place	Explanation
1930	70	F	Yakama	Heart Trouble
1930	70	M	Yakama	Heart Trouble
1931	65	M	Yakama	Endocarditis
1931	62	M	Yakama	Heart Disease
1931	0	M	Yakama	Heart Disease/Died at Birth
1931	37	F	Yakama	Heart Disease and Goiter
1931	37	F	Yakama	Goiter and Septic Heart
1931	65	M	Yakama	Chronic Endocarditis
1932	43	M	Off Rez	Heart Disease
1934	41	F	Off Rez	Heart Failure Following Hysterectomy
1935	49	F	Yakama	Heart Disease/Nephritis
1935	49	F	Yakama	Aortic and Mitral Insufficiency
1936	49	F	Yakama	Heart Disease/Jaundice
1936	50	M	Yakama	Heart Disease
1936	71	F	Yakama	Heart Disease
1936	58	M	Yakama	Heart Disease
1936	—	F	Yakama	Heart Disease/Adult
1936	95	F	Yakama	Heart Disease With Rheumatism
1936	99	M	Off Rez	Arteriosclerosis/Second-Degree Burns
1936	80	F	Yakama	Heart Disease
1936	71	F	Yakama	Heart Disease
1936	60	M	Yakama	Heart Disease
1936	80	F	Yakama	Heart Disease
1936	58	M	Yakama	Heart Disease
1937	84	F	Off Rez	Arteriosclerosis
1937	38	M	Off Rez	Heart Disease/Pleurisy
1937	79	F	Yakama	Heart Disease
1937	84	F	Off Rez	Arteriosclerosis
1938	68	M	Off Rez	Heart Disease
1938	86	M	Yakama	Heart Disease/Natural Causes
1938	90	M	Off Rez	Heart Disease/Nephritis
1938	62	M	Yakama	Heart Disease
1938	66	F	Yakama	Heart Disease
1938	68	M	Off Rez	Heart Disease
1938	65	F	Yakama	Heart Disease
1938	66	F	Yakama	Heart Disease
1938	86	M	Yakama	Heart Disease
1939	77	F	Yakama	Heart Disease/Bronchitis

Year	Age	Gender	Place	Explanation
1939	56	M	Yakama	Heart Disease
1939	81	M	Yakama	Heart Disease
1939	63	F	Off Rez	Heart Disease
1939	76	M	Yakama	Heart Disease/Natural Causes
1939	79	M	Off Rez	Heart Disease
1939	71	M	Yakama	Heart Disease
1939	56	M	Yakama	Heart Disease
1939	76	M	Yakama	Heart Disease/Natural Causes
1939	79	M	Off Rez	Heart Disease
1939	81	M	Yakama	Heart Disease
1939	62	M	Yakama	Heart Disease
1939	77	F	Yakama	Heart Disease/Pulmonary Disease
1939	77	F	Off Rez	Heart Disease
1940	28	F	Off Rez	Heart Disease
1940	48	M	Yakama	Pulmonary Edema
1940	77	F	Off Rez	Arteriosclerosis/Pneumonia
1940	49	F	Off Rez	Heart Disease
1940	41	M	Yakama	Heart Disease
1940	41	M	Yakama	Heart Disease
1940	28	F	Off Rez	Heart Disease
1940	49	F	Off Rez	Heart Disease
1941	81	F	Hospital	Heart Disease
1941	54	F	Off Rez	Heart Disease
1941	36	F	Yakama	Pulmonary Embolism
1941	90	F	Yakama	Heart Disease
1941	0	F	Yakama	Heart Disease
1941	58	F	Yakama	Heart Disease
1941	76	M	Yakama	Heart Disease
1941	22	M	Yakama	Pulmonary Hemorrhage
1941	36	F	Yakama	Pulmonary Embolism/Heart Disease
1941	58	F	Yakama	Heart Disease
1941	22	M	Yakama	Pulmonary Hemorrhage
1941	0	F	Yakama	Heart Disease/Diarrhea
1941	90	F	Yakama	Heart Disease/Natural Causes
1941	76	M	Yakama	Heart Disease/Syphilis
1942	12	M	Yakama	Heart Disease
1942	48	M	Yakama	Heart Disease and Nephritis
1942	84	F	Yakama	Heart Disease
1942	90	F	Yakama	Heart Disease

Year	Age	Gender	Place	Explanation
1942	71	M	Off Rez	Heart Disease
1942	81	M	Yakama	Heart Disease and Syphilis
1942	12	F	Yakama	Heart Disease
1942	48	M	Yakama	Heart Disease/Nephritis
1942	84	F	Yakama	Circulatory Failure/Heart Disease
1942	12	F	Yakama	Heart Disease/Tonsillitis
1943	68	F	Off Rez	Heart Disease
1943	68	M	Off Rez	Heart Disease
1943	9	F	Off Rez	Pulmonary Hemorrhage
1943	64	M	Yakama	Pulmonary Ederose/Luetic
1943	55	F	Yakama	Heart Disease
1943	38	M	Off Rez	Heart Disease
1943	81	F	Yakama	Heart Disease
1943	68	M	Yakama	Heart Disease
1943	58	F	Yakama	Heart Disease
1943	54	F	Yakama	Heart Disease
1943	0	F	Yakama	Heart Disease
1943	99	M	Yakama	Heart Disease and Natural Causes
1943	52	F	Yakama	Heart Disease
1943	64	M	Yakama	Pulmonary Edema and Heart Disease
1943	99	F	Yakama	Heart Disease
1943	68	F	Off Rez	Heart Disease
1943	75	F	Yakama	Heart Disease
1943	54	F	Yakama	Heart Disease
1944	56	F	Yakama	Heart Disease
1944	55	—	Off Rez	Heart Disease
1944	53	F	Yakama	Heart Disease
1944	77	F	Yakama	Heart Disease/Abdominal Tumor
1944	90	F	Off Rez	Heart Disease
1944	0	F	Yakama	Heart Disease
1944	77	F	Yakama	Heart Disease
1944	86	F	Yakama	Heart Disease/Natural Causes
1944	68	F	Yakama	Heart Disease
1944	0	F	Yakama	Heart Disease
1944	75	F	Yakama	Heart Disease
1944	54	F	Yakama	Heart Disease
1945	5	F	Yakama	Heart Disease
1945	70	M	Yakama	Heart Disease
1945	61	M	Off Rez	Heart Disease

Year	Age	Gender	Place	Explanation
1945	29	F	Off Rez	Heart Disease
1945	54	M	Yakama	Heart Disease
1945	50	F	Off Rez	Heart Disease
1945	76	F	Yakama	Heart Disease
1945	54	M	Yakama	Heart Disease
1945	72	M	Off Rez	Heart Disease
1945	75	F	Yakama	Heart Disease
1945	14	M	Yakama	Pulmonary Edema
1945	39	F	Yakama	Heart Disease
1946	65	F	Off Rez	Heart Disease
1946	67	M	Off Rez	Heart Disease
1946	1	M	Yakama	Heart Disease
1946	81	F	Yakama	Heart Disease
1946	49	M	Off Rez	Heart Disease
1946	79	F	Yakama	Heart Disease
1946	57	M	Yakama	Heart Disease
1947	81	F	Off Rez	Heart Disease
1947	45	F	Off Rez	Heart Disease
1947	4	F	Off Rez	Heart Disease
1947	0	F	Yakama	Heart Disease
1947	75	F	Off Rez	Heart Disease
1947	46	M	Yakama	Heart Disease
1947	0	F	Yakama	Heart Disease
1947	74	M	Yakama	Heart Disease
1947	74	F	Off Rez	Heart Disease/Burns from Fire
1947	0	M	Yakama	Heart Disease/Premature Childbirth
1948	75	M	Yakama	Heart Disease
1948	58	F	Yakama	Heart Disease
1948	88	M	Yakama	Heart Disease
1948	50	F	Off Rez	Heart Disease
1948	41	F	Off Rez	Heart Disease
1948	90	F	Off Rez	Heart Disease/Natural Causes
1948	48	M	Off Rez	Pulmonary Edema/Heart Failure
1949	70	F	Off Rez	Heart Disease
1949	76	F	Off Rez	Heart Disease
1949	80	F	Off Rez	Natural Causes/Heart Failure
1949	58	M	Off Rez	Heart Disease
1949	63	M	Yakama	Heart Disease
1949	10	M	Yakama	Heart Disease

Year	Age	Gender	Place	Explanation
1949	0	M	Yakama	Heart Disease
1949	63	F	Yakama	Heart Disease
1949	79	M	Yakama	Heart Disease
1950	75	F	Off Rez	Heart Disease
1950	71	M	Yakama	Heart Disease
1950	57	F	Off Rez	Arteriosclerosis
1950	43	F	Yakama	Heart Disease
1950	48	F	Yakama	Heart Disease
1951	39	F	Yakama	Pernicious Anemia/Endocarditis
1951	32	M	Off Rez	Heart Disease
1951	62	F	Yakama	Heart Disease/Pneumonia
1952	72	F	Yakama	Heart Disease
1952	1	F	Yakama	Heart Disease
1952	62	M	Yakama	Heart Disease
1952	29	F	Yakama	Heart Disease
1952	63	M	Yakama	Heart Disease
1952	80	F	Yakama	Heart Disease
1952	83	M	Yakama	Heart Disease
1953	94	F	Yakama	Heart Disease
1953	70	F	Yakama	Heart Disease/Syphilis
1953	84	F	Yakama	Heart Disease
1953	66	F	Off Rez	Heart Disease
1953	67	M	Off Rez	Heart Disease
1953	73	M	Yakama	Heart Disease
1953	74	M	Yakama	Heart Disease
1953	62	M	Off Rez	Pulmonary Embolism
1953	47	M	Yakama	Heart Disease
1954	65	F	Yakama	Acute Myocardial Infarction
1954	90	M	Yakama	Arteriosclerosis
1954	70	F	Off Rez	Heart Disease
1954	78	M	Yakama	Signs of Senility/Heart Attack
1954	45	F	Yakama	Signs of Heart Attack
1954	67	F	Yakama	Myocardial Thrombosis
1954	77	F	Yakama	Signs of Coronary Attack
1954	68	M	Off Rez	Probably Chronic Myocarditis
1954	34	F	Yakama	Arteriosclerosis
1954	—	M	Yakama	Heart Lesion
1954	73	M	Yakama	Heart Lesion
1954	72	F	Yakama	Coronary Attack/Senility
1955	56	M	Off Rez	Cerebral Vascular Hypertension

Year	Age	Gender	Place	Explanation
1955	72	M	Yakama	Coronary Occlusion
1955	65	M	Yakama	Coronary Occlusion
1955	0	F	Yakama	Toxic Myocarditis
1955	63	M	Yakama	Acute Myocardial Infarction
1955	67	M	Yakama	Signs of Heart Attack
1955	72	M	Yakama	Signs of Coronary Attack
1955	55	M	Off Rez	Myocardial Infarction
1955	53	F	Off Rez	Cardiac Failure/Cervix Carcinoma
1955	67	F	Off Rez	Cardiac Failure, Myocardial Related
1955	65	F	Yakama	Signs of Coronary Attack
1955	85	M	Yakama	Possibly Chronic Myocarditis
1955	99	F	Yakama	Probably Myocardial Failure
1955	64	M	Yakama	Signs of Coronary Attack
1955	45	M	Off Rez	Coronary Occlusion
1955	39	F	Yakama	Coronary Occlusion
1955	80	F	Yakama	Coronary Thrombosis
1955	60	M	Yakama	Coronary Occlusion/ Arteriosclerosis
1956	61	M	Yakama	Signs of Coronary Attack
1956	56	M	Off Rez	Coronary Occlusion/ Arteriosclerosis
1956	88	M	Off Rez	Possibly Chronic Myocarditis
1957	65	F	Off Rez	Cardiac Failure/Arteriosclerosis
1957	77	M	Off Rez	Uremia/Nephritis/Arteriosclerosis
1957	72	M	Yakama	Heart Block, Arteriosclerotic
1957	44	M	Yakama	Probably Myocardial Failure
1957	56	F	Off Rez	Pulmonary Edema, Cardiac
1958	62	M	Yakama	Signs of Heart Attack
1958	72	M	Off Rez	Myocardial Failure,Heart Disease
1958	62	M	Yakama	Acute Myocardial Infarction
1958	88	F	Off Rez	Vascular Accident/Arteriosclerosis
1958	95	M	Off Rez	Vascular Accident/Arteriosclerosis
1958	99	M	Yakama	Myocarditis/Arteriosclerosis
1958	65	M	Off Rez	Coronary Heart Disease
1958	42	M	Off Rez	Chronic Rheumatic Heart Disease
1958	58	M	Yakama	Signs of Heart Attack
1958	70	F	Off Rez	Heart Failure/Myocarditis
1958	78	M	Off Rez	Myocardial Infarction
1959	70	M	Yakama	Congestive Heart Failure

Year	Age	Gender	Place	Explanation
1959	93	F	Yakama	Signs of Heart Attack
1959	74	M	Off Rez	Coronary Occlusion
1959	53	M	Yakama	Signs of Heart Attack
1959	0	M	Off Rez	Pulmonary Obstruction
1959	51	F	Off Rez	Cardiac Insufficiency
1959	38	F	Off Rez	Chronic Myocarditis
1959	44	M	Off Rez	Acute Myocardial Infarction
1959	64	F	Yakama	Myocardial Thrombosis/ Alcoholism
1960	43	M	Yakama	Heart Failure/Alcoholism
1960	63	F	Off Rez	Myocarditis/Nephritis
1960	71	F	Off Rez	Myocardial Failure
1960	58	M	Off Rez	Probably Myocardial Infarction
1960	64	F	Hospital	Probably Myocardial Infarction
1960	99	F	Hospital	Cardiac Arrest
1960	78	M	Off Rez	Chronic Myocarditis
1960	58	F	Off Rez	Heart Disease/Arteriosclerosis
1960	74	M	Off Rez	Myocardial Infarction
1961	86	F	Off Rez	Coronary Occlusion/ Arteriosclerosis
1961	58	M	Off Rez	Pulmonary Edema, Myocardial
1961	79	F	Hospital	Cardiac Arrest/Myocardial Infarction
1961	84	F	Off Rez	Coronary Heart Disease/ Arteriosclerosis
1961	71	M	Off Rez	Cardiac and Respiratory Failure
1961	56	M	Hospital	Coronary Thrombosis/ Arteriosclerosis
1961	69	M	Off Rez	Myocardial Infarction
1962	43	M	Off Rez	Coronary Insufficiency/ Arteriosclerosis
1962	68	F	Off Rez	Cerebral Vascular Accident/ Arteriosclerosis
1962	99	F	Off Rez	Arteriosclerosis/Carcinoma
1962	0	M	Off Rez	Heart Failure/Bronchiolitis
1962	69	M	Off Rez	Cardiac Arrest
1962	45	M	Off Rez	Heart Failure/Pulmonary Complications
1962	44	M	Hospital	Probably Chronic Heart Disease

Year	Age	Gender	Place	Explanation
1962	74	F	Off Rez	Arrhythmia/Thrombosis/ Arteriosclerosis
1962	99	M	Hospital	Heart Failure/ASHD
1963	89	F	Off Rez	Cardiac Failure/ASCVD
1963	99	F	Off Rez	Myocardial Failure/Arteriosclerosis
1963	83	F	Hospital	Coronary Insufficiency/ Arteriosclerosis
1963	71	M	Hospital	Signs of Heart Attack
1963	84	F	Off Rez	Coronary Thrombosis
1963	0	M	Off Rez	Congenital Heart Disease
1963	86	M	Off Rez	Heart Disease
1963	62	F	Off Rez	Hemorrhage/Cardiovascular Disease
1963	66	M	Off Rez	Cerebral Thrombosis/ Arteriosclerosis
1963	1	M	Off Rez	Edema/Cardiac Failure/ Fibroelastosis
1964	63	F	Off Rez	Myocardial Infarction
1964	0	M	Off Rez	Cardiac Arrest
1964	93	F	Off Rez	Coronary Infarction/ Arteriosclerosis
1964	85	F	Off Rez	Arteriosclerotic Disease
1964	25	M	Hospital	Signs of Heart Attack
1964	56	M	Hospital	Signs of Heart Attack

Gastrointestinal Disorders

TODAY IT IS DIFFICULT TO CONCEIVE of a time when gastrointestinal disorders caused so many deaths, but before 1950 and the development of antibiotics, many maladies of the stomach and intestines killed people, particularly children and elders. On the Yakama Reservation, gastrointestinal disorders killed 124 people between 1888 and 1964. Although the digestive tract naturally contains vital bacteria, dangerous bacteria can spread within the digestive tract, causing illnesses and deaths. People ingested bacteria that came into contact with the gut wall and circulated within the body through the blood stream. Unwashed hands and fingers contributed to the ingestion of bacteria, but mothers could unwittingly infect their infants and babies by feeding them with unclean breasts or contaminated bottles. Furthermore, infants and children also infected themselves with bacteria by touching soil, dust, or fecal material infused with bacteria or viruses that could enter their bodies through their mouths. By coincidentally touching the excrement of infected people, caretakers could spread the malady to themselves and others, especially if they prepared food, handled dishes, or used their unclean fingers to touch and probe patients. In a world unfamiliar with pathogens, diseases could spread rapidly within a family through normal nursing of sick individuals. This does not suggest that Yakama were filthy people or that they carelessly functioned in their world. Rather, like many people of the late 19th and early 20th centuries, Yakama people simply did not know about the existence of bacteria and did not have knowledge of public health, a budding movement among non-Indians. Public health was slowly introduced to reservations through Indian schools, field nurses, and medical doctors, but these conditions of public health developed very slowly on reservations because of the lack of funding provided by Congress and the Office of Indian Affairs. Prior to the reservation system, Yakama people had lived in permanent villages, but they moved about a great deal during the course of the year from hunting to gathering to fishing grounds. Each time they moved, Indian women cleaned their camps and cared for their bedding. However, with the creation of reservations, people spent more and more time living in one location and in one house, unable to dismantle their homes or villages and care for each other in the manner known in the past. Furthermore, the reservation system became the space where new pathogens met vulnerable hosts. Bacteria and viruses opportunistically found new hosts. On reservations, microorganisms found weakened and vulnerable bodies that provided a new source of life for pathogens and death for their hosts. In some cases, people became ill with a form of gastrointestinal disease that caused a variety of symptoms.

Children and adults infected with gastrointestinal diseases exhibited one or more of these symptoms. Some of them experienced general discomfort in the stomach or intestines, much like contemporary people do when they have stomach aches. However, the pain could become progressively worse from severe cramps that doubled up victims and made them cry out in pain. A person suffering from a gastrointestinal disorder could experience vomiting and diarrhea, which could prove dangerous to a Yakama person due to the loss of vital body fluids. A state of dehydration could further threaten the lives of people, particularly among infants and small children who could not live long in a dehydrated state. Agency officials recorded that most died of "entero colitis," "intestinal infection," "acute gastro enteritis," and "stomach trouble." Other children died of "diarrhea," "infantile dysentery," "dehydration from enteritis," and "convulsions from gastroenteritis." Sometimes, agents writing the descriptions of deaths on the reservation stated that causes included "bowel trouble," "intestinal obstruction," or "choleliathiasis." Today, the significance of gastrointestinal disorders has greatly declined, although medical professionals still teach parents about the dangers of bacteria and viruses as well as the deadly consequences of dehydration within an infant's body. Although gastrointestinal disorders are no longer the killer they once were, they remain a real threat to the lives of infants and children on the reservations.

Year	Age	Gender	Place	Explanation
1924	30	F	Yakama	Stomach Trouble
1924	80	M	Yakama	Chronic Dysentery/Old Age
1924	44	F	Yakama	Acute Indigestion
1924	61	F	Yakama	Acute Indigestion
1925	0	F	Yakama	Stomach Trouble
1925	0	M	Yakama	Enterocolitis
1925	3	M	Yakama	Enteritis
1925	1	F	Yakama	Bowel Trouble
1925	3	M	Yakama	Bowel Trouble
1925	2	M	Yakama	Stomach Trouble
1927	1	F	Yakama	Ptomaine
1927	1	M	Yakama	Dysentery
1927	0	F	Yakama	Enterocolitis
1927	1	F	Yakama	Ptomaine
1927	0	F	Yakama	Enterocolitis
1927	1	M	Yakama	Dysentery
1927	57	F	Yakama	Intestinal Obstruction
1928	0	F	Off Rez	Gastroenteritis
1928	0	F	Off Rez	Gastroenteritis
1928	34	F	Off Rez	Acute Indigestion/Influenza
1929	1	M	Yakama	Illium Involved Problem
1929	0	M	Yakama	Acute Gastroenteritis
1929	0	M	Yakama	Acute Gastroenteritis
1929	1	M	Off Rez	Intusseption of Ileum
1930	0	F	Yakama	Enterocolitis
1930	0	F	Yakama	Enterocolitis
1930	4	F	Off Rez	Gastroenteritis
1930	1	F	Yakama	Enterocolitis
1930	3	F	Off Rez	Gastroenteritis
1931	0	F	Yakama	Intestinal Infection
1931	0	F	Yakama	Intestinal Infection
1933	0	M	Off Rez	Diarrhea
1933	34	F	Yakama	Choleliathiasis
1933	0	M	Yakama	Diarrhea
1934	70	F	Yakama	Intestinal Problems/Nephritis
1935	4	M	Yakama	Gastroenteritis
1935	4	M	Yakama	Gastroenteritis
1937	5	F	Yakama	Ileocolitis/Dehydration
1937	0	F	Yakama	Diarrhea
1937	0	F	Yakama	Enterocolitis

Year	Age	Gender	Place	Explanation
1937	0	M	Yakama	Diarrhea/Pneumonia
1937	5	F	Yakama	Ileocolitis
1937	0	F	Yakama	Enterocolitis
1938	87	M	Yakama	Bowel Obstruction
1938	0	F	Yakama	Gastroenteritis
1938	1	F	Yakama	Infantile Dysentery
1938	87	M	Yakama	Bowel Obstruction
1939	0	F	Off Rez	Dysentery
1939	0	M	Yakama	Infantile Dysentery
1939	1	M	Off Rez	Dysentery
1939	0	M	Yakama	Enterocolitis/Pneumonia
1939	0	M	Yakama	Infantile Dysentery
1940	0	M	Yakama	Gastroenteritis
1940	2	M	Yakama	Gastroenteritis
1940	0	F	Yakama	Enteritis
1940	1	M	Yakama	Dysentery
1940	0	F	Yakama	Gastroenteritis/Malnutrition
1940	1	F	Yakama	Gastroenteritis
1940	4	M	Yakama	Gastroenteritis
1940	1	M	Yakama	Dysentery
1940	0	F	Yakama	Epidemic
1940	0	F	Yakama	Enteritis
1940	2	M	Yakama	Gastroenteritis
1940	1	M	Yakama	Gastroenteritis
1940	1	F	Yakama	Gastroenteritis
1940	0	F	Yakama	Diarrhea
1940	2	M	Off Rez	Gastroenteritis
1941	0	F	Yakama	Gastroenteritis/Pneumonia
1941	76	F	Yakama	Gastroenteritis
1941	0	F	Yakama	Gastroenteritis
1941	0	F	Off Rez	Enteritis
1941	1	F	Yakama	Gastroenteritis/Pneumonia
1941	0	M	Yakama	Enteritis
1941	76	F	Off Rez	Gastroenteritis/Heart Disease
1941	0	M	Yakama	Enteritis
1941	1	F	Yakama	Gastroenteritis/Pneumonia
1941	77	F	Yakama	Gastroenteritis/Heart Disease
1941	0	M	Yakama	Enteritis
1942	1	M	Yakama	Gastroenteritis/Diabetes
1942	0	M	Yakama	Dysentery

Year	Age	Gender	Place	Explanation
1943	0	M	Yakama	Dysentery
1943	5	M	Off Rez	Gastroenteritis
1943	69	F	Yakama	Intestinal Obstruction/Colitis
1943	16	F	Off Rez	Gastroenteritis
1944	0	F	Yakama	Dysentery
1944	1	M	Off Rez	Diarrhea/Enteritis/Pneumonia
1944	1	M	Off Rez	Gastroenteritis
1944	0	M	Yakama	Diarrhea
1944	0	F	Yakama	Dysentery
1944	0	F	Yakama	Enteritis with Dehydration
1944	1	M	Yakama	Dehydration from Enteritis
1945	0	F	Yakama	Convulsions from Gastroenteritis
1945	0	F	Yakama	Dysentery
1945	0	M	Off Rez	Enteritis
1945	1	M	Yakama	Gastroenteritis
1948	0	M	Yakama	Diarrhea
1949	0	M	Off Rez	Gastroenteritis
1952	1	M	Off Rez	Diarrhea/Rickets
1952	0	F	Yakama	Diarrhea/Possibly Syphilis
1952	1	M	Off Rez	Gastroenteritis
1954	0	M	Off Rez	Enteritis/Acidosis/Otitis Media
1954	0	M	Off Rez	Acidosis Enteritis
1954	0	F	Off Rez	Acute Enteritis
1954	0	M	Off Rez	Acute Enteritis
1955	0	M	Off Rez	Diarrhea/Nephritis/Myocardia
1955	0	F	Off Rez	Acute Gastroenteritis
1955	0	F	Off Rez	Infectious Diarrhea
1956	0	M	Off Rez	Diarrhea/Pneumonia
1957	0	M	Off Rez	Toxic Illeus/Diarrhea
1957	0	F	Off Rez	Dehydration/Acute Enteritis
1958	0	F	Off Rez	Diarrhea
1958	0	F	Off Rez	Dehydration/Gastroenteritis
1958	0	F	Off Rez	Diarrhea
1958	0	M	Off Rez	Acute Gastroenteritis
1958	1	F	Off Rez	Acute Gastroenteritis
1961	0	M	Off Rez	Infectious Diarrhea
1961	25	M	Hospital	Viral Gastroenteritis
1962	0	M	—	Dehydration/Diarrhea
1962	0	M	Off Rez	Gastroenteritis
1962	0	F	Off Rez	Infectious Diarrhea

Year	Age	Gender	Place	Explanation
1962	0	F	Hospital	Dehydration/Diarrhea
1963	1	M	Off Rez	Diarrhea/Anemia/Malnutrition
1964	1	F	Off Rez	Gastroenteritis
1964	3	F	Off Rez	Acute Enteritis

Influenza

HISTORICALLY, INFLUENZA HAS BEEN A DANGEROUS and deceptive disease that mutates, thus making it difficult to fight. Eighteenth-century Italians believed that the stars controlled such diseases and that influenza was a part of the astrological cycle. As a result, they named it "influence," thus influenza. The French called the disease "grippe," but contemporary American society labeled the disease "flu," simply a shortened version of influenza. The disease may have been present for a thousand or more years, but in 1510, European chroniclers provided the first full description of influenza. It likely appeared first in Africa, Europe, and Asia, moving out from these hubs to other worlds, including Native America. Influenza likely emerged from those populations that domesticated birds and animals, including pigs, cattle, chickens, ducks, and other animals. Humans and animals pass influenza viruses back and forth, sharing the ambitious pathogens. In fact, humans may share viruses with undomesticated birds, and the viruses often travel great distances in unsuspecting hosts. In the 18th century, Europe experienced five pandemics of influenza, the worst of which occurred in 1781 and 1782, at the end of the American Revolution. Although British soldiers and sailors had been regularly inoculated for smallpox (unlike American troops), they had no vaccine for the influenza viruses.

As a result of the Revolutionary War, travel, and trade, influenza spread in the United States during the early Federalist period. The growth of the American population, immigration, farming development, expansionism, and other factors contributed to numerous Americans dying of influenza in the 1830s, including an unknown number of American Indians. In 1889 and 1890, influenza struck the United States again, bringing illness and death. Then the disease remained relatively constant during the 1890s and early 20th century until 1918, when it exploded. Wars throughout the world may have contributed to the great pandemic of influenza of 1918 to 1919, because conflicts in Russia, South Africa, and China required the movement of large numbers of troops, supplies, and civilians to many corners of the world. By 1918, even the United States had become involved in the Great War, and the terrible influenza pandemic, often called the Spanish Influenza, emerged in the United States. Initially, in 1918, a mild form of influenza infected many people throughout the world, but by August the disease mutated into a killer virus. It appeared to emerge in three places at the same time, West Africa, Western France, and Boston, Massachusetts. All three areas featured ports that handled thousands of troops and supplies to the western front. From these three points, influenza spread to all quarters of the globe, including Indian America. By 1918 to 1919, the bodies and immune systems of Yakama Indians had been compromised by changes in diets, the lack of health providers, the absence of major public health service, inadequate housing, and anomie.

In 1918 and 1919, some youngsters on the Yakama Reservation attending government or church schools must have heard and repeated the popular song "I had a little bird. And its name was Enza. I opened the window. And influenza." The influenza virus of 1918 killed 17 Yakama people on the reservation, and two the next year. The insidious disease killed Yakama people in subsequent years but never again that many. Still in 1924, 11 people lost their lives to influenza and the next year, 10 Yakamas died of the dreadful disease. In 1928, 15 people passed away due to influenza, making that year a significant one in terms of influenza deaths on the reservation. The number of deaths caused by influenza declined after 1928, but as late as 1962, a female infant died of the dreadful disease, accompanied by meningitis. Like elsewhere in the world, the influenza epidemic of 1918 on the Yakama Reservation took the lives of those individuals in the prime of their lives, those between 20 and 40 years of age. On the reservation, this age group suffered ten deaths, while teenagers experienced four deaths. Only three people over forty years of age died in 1918, because of flu, and only one infant, a male, died that year. Clearly, young people—working people of marrying and childbearing age—suffered the most from the influenza virus of 1918. Influenza was only one of many maladies that preyed on the bodies of Yakama people, but for certain years, it was a prominent killer.

Year	Age	Gender	Place	Explanation
1918	68	M	Yakama	Grippe (Influenza)
1918	57	M	Yakama	Spanish Influenza/Tuberculosis
1918	45	M	Yakama	Spanish Influenza/Tuberculosis
1918	39	M	Yakama	Spanish Influenza
1918	33	M	Yakama	Spanish Influenza
1918	26	F	Yakama	Spanish Influenza
1918	16	F	Yakama	Spanish Influenza/Tuberculosis
1918	16	F	Yakama	Spanish Influenza/Tuberculosis
1918	30	M	Yakama	Spanish Influenza/Tuberculosis
1918	1	M	Yakama	Spanish Influenza
1918	34	M	Yakama	Spanish Influenza
1918	34	F	Yakama	Spanish Influenza
1918	28	F	Yakama	Influenza
1918	13	F	Yakama	Spanish Influenza
1918	15	M	Yakama	Spanish Influenza
1918	31	M	Yakama	Influenza
1918	36	F	Yakama	Spanish Influenza
1919	17	M	Yakama	Spanish Influenza
1919	29	F	Yakama	Influenza
1920	21	F	Yakama	Influenza/Pneumonia
1922	41	F	Yakama	Influenza/Pneumonia
1924	89	F	Yakama	Influenza
1924	78	M	Yakama	Influenza
1924	50	F	Yakama	Influenza
1924	3	M	Yakama	Influenza
1924	56	F	Yakama	Influenza
1924	6	F	Yakama	Influenza
1924	61	F	Yakama	Influenza
1924	69	M	Yakama	Grippe/Influenza
1924	50	F	Yakama	Influenza
1924	6	M	Yakama	Influenza
1924	56	F	Yakama	Influenza
1925	61	M	Yakama	Influenza
1925	48	F	Yakama	Influenza
1925	65	M	Yakama	Old Age/Influenza
1925	73	F	Yakama	Influenza
1925	48	F	Yakama	Influenza
1925	85	M	Yakama	Influenza
1925	70	F	Yakama	Old Age/Influenza
1925	9	M	Yakama	Influenza

Year	Age	Gender	Place	Explanation
1925	78	M	Yakama	Old Age/Influenza
1925	8	M	Yakama	Influenza
1926	8	M	Yakama	Influenza
1926	70	F	Yakama	Influenza
1926	8	M	Yakama	Influenza
1926	85	M	Yakama	Influenza
1926	85	M	Yakama	Influenza
1927	64	F	Yakama	Influenza
1927	75	F	Yakama	Influenza
1927	55	F	Yakama	Influenza
1927	75	F	Yakama	Influenza
1927	55	F	Yakama	Influenza
1927	28	F	Yakama	Influenza
1927	64	F	Yakama	Influenza
1927	40	F	Yakama	—
1928	57	M	Yakama	Influenza
1928	84	M	Yakama	Influenza
1928	12	M	Yakama	Influenza
1928	56	M	Yakama	Influenza
1928	64	F	Yakama	Influenza
1928	6	M	Yakama	Influenza
1928	78	M	Yakama	Influenza
1928	75	M	Yakama	Influenza
1928	6	M	Yakama	—
1928	75	M	Yakama	—
1928	0	M	Off Rez	Intestinal Influenza
1928	88	F	Off Rez	Influenza
1928	69	M	Off Rez	Senility/Influenza
1928	64	F	Off Rez	Influenza
1928	74	F	Off Rez	Influenza
1929	74	M	Yakama	—
1929	72	F	Yakama	—
1929	23	M	Off Rez	—
1929	74	F	Yakama	—
1929	72	F	Yakama	Influenza/Senility
1929	6	M	Yakama	Influenza
1929	80	F	Yakama	Old Age/Influenza
1929	22	F	Yakama	Septic Sore Throat/Influenza
1931	64	F	Off Rez	Influenza
1931	4	F	Yakama	Influenza

Year	Age	Gender	Place	Explanation
1931	64	F	Yakama	Influenza
1931	31	F	Yakama	Influenza/Bronchopneumonia
1931	57	M	Yakama	Influenza
1931	0	F	Yakama	Influenza
1932	79	F	Yakama	Influenza
1932	88	F	Yakama	Influenza
1932	88	F	Yakama	Influenza
1932	79	F	Yakama	Influenza
1934	26	M	Yakama	Influenza
1937	85	F	Yakama	Influenza
1937	67	M	Yakama	Influenza
1937	75	F	Off Rez	Influenza/Choleliathiasis
1937	67	M	Off Rez	Influenza
1937	75	F	Off Rez	Influenza
1940	58	F	Yakama	Influenza
1940	48	M	Yakama	Influenza
1940	58	F	Yakama	Influenza
1944	0	F	Yakama	Influenza with Otitis Media
1944	0	F	Yakama	Influenza/Complications
1953	0	M	Yakama	Influenza since Birth
1953	99	F	Off Rez	Influenza
1956	51	F	Yakama	Influenza/Pulmonary Tuberculosis
1959	65	M	Off Rez	Influenza
1962	0	F	Off Rez	Influenza/Meningitis

Cancer

CELLS INFECTED BY CANCER experience unregulated growth. The disease can develop in any organ and within any tissue. When cancer cells grow, they can multiply, forming a mass of cancerous tissue that attacks surrounding normal tissues. When cells and tissues move to healthy cells and tissue, specialist call this process "metastasizing." This causes cancer to spread. Thus, cancer cells emerge from normal cells, a complex process called transformation. A change in the cell prior to this change takes place, and medical scholars call this process "initiation." As a result of initiation and transformation, the cell's genetic material (DNA) changes, and this process occurs because of a carcinogen, or an agent such as radiation, chemicals, viruses, or sunlight is introduced. A genetic flaw in a cell may "promote" or make the cell more susceptible to cancer. Thus, several factors contribute to the onslaught of cancer. Once cancer develops in a cell, the body's immune system attacks the cancer, destroying it before it can fully develop and grow. When a person's immune system becomes compromised by ill health, malnutrition, stress, viruses, or other factors, the immune system often cannot destroy the cancer. This was the case for many Native Americans during the 19th and early 20th centuries.

Before the 1920s, few documents existed about cancer cases and deaths on the Yakama Reservation. As a result, it is impossible to discover if family history had any influence on cancer deaths after 1925, when agents first recorded a death caused by cancer. Furthermore, it is impossible to determine to what extent the Hanford Nuclear Power Plant may have contributed historically to cancer deaths on the Yakama Reservation. While it is certain that atomic radiation contributes to increased cases of cancer, the health effects of the power plant among Yakama people between the 1940s and 1960s cannot be ascertained from these data. Today, scientists understand that pesticides also can contribute to cancers, but no measurement has been attempted to assess the historical significance of pesticides during the early 20th century within the Yakima Valley. However, cases of death caused by radiation, pesticides, and other likely contributors of cancer deaths are not noted in this data set.

Today, scholars also know that diets high in fiber contribute to fewer cases of cancers originating in the gastrointestinal tract. Before the 1950s, most Yakama had enjoyed diets high in fiber provided by natural fruits and vegetables, particularly the numerous roots once consumed by the people. In addition, they once had eaten large quantities of salmon and other fish, some of which had been smoked (a contributing factor in cancer), but most of which was eaten fresh or dried on racks like jerky. With the arrival of non-Indians in the Inland Northwest and the creation of the reservation system, Indians had fewer opportunities to travel to gathering areas. In addition, non-Indian soldiers, government officials, ferrymen, farmers, ranchers, merchants, and others took over former Indian lands where the people had hunted, fished, and gathered. Conflicts over ownership and use of such areas emerged, and during the years under examination, Yakama people had more difficulty obtaining native foods. Today, scientists know that when the immune system is suppressed, the body is more vulnerable to diseases, including cancer. Thus, as a result of physical and psychological consequences, Yakama people became more susceptible to cancers of all sorts.

Yakama people died from many types of cancer. In 1925, the Office of Indian Affairs recorded the first death resulting from cancer, a woman, 50 years old, who died of stomach cancer. From 1925 to 1964, 11 people died of stomach cancer, one of foremost causes of cancer deaths. A total of four people died of lung cancer, suggesting that it was not a marked cause of cancer deaths, perhaps in part because tobacco use among Yakama people had not reached a critical point. Before World War II, some Yakama had used tobacco but the number of cigarette smokers likely increased due to the war and radio, television, motion picture, and print advertisements during the war and postwar period. Yakama people also died of cancers of the brain, intestine, rectum, and bladder. However, females suffered the most pronounced forms of cancer among the Yakama, including breast cancer and reproductive cancers. A total of 23 women died of a carcinoma connected to their reproductive systems, including uterine, cervical, and ovarian cancers. Reproduction cancers among Yakama women constituted the largest number of deaths by any single cancer, and women suffered 71 percent (n = 58) of all cancer deaths. Perhaps papillomavirus, which causes genital warts, contributed to causing so much reproductive cancer among women.

Year	Age	Gender	Place	Explanation
1925	50	F	Yakama	Cancer of Stomach
1925	68	M	Yakama	Carcinoma
1925	56	F	Yakama	Liver Carcinoma
1925	56	F	Yakama	Liver Carcinoma
1926	72	F	Yakama	Liver Carcinoma
1928	83	F	Yakama	Cancer
1928	65	F	Off Rez	Uterine Cancer
1928	83	F	Yakama	Cancer
1929	55	F	Yakama	Cancer of Stomach
1929	55	F	Yakama	Cancer of Stomach
1929	63	F	Yakama	Cancer of Cervix
1929	63	F	Yakama	Cancer of Cervix
1931	13	F	Yakama	Cancer of Stomach
1931	47	F	Off Rez	Breast Cancer
1931	69	M	Off Rez	Cancer
1931	67	F	Yakama	Cancer
1931	67	F	Yakama	Cancer of the Stomach
1933	62	F	Yakama	Uterine Cancer
1933	62	F	Hospital	Uterine Carcinoma
1934	37	F	Off Rez	Fat Embolus/Uterine Cancer
1935	60	F	Yakama	Uterine Cancer
1935	60	F	Yakama	Uterine Carcinoma
1939	68	F	Yakama	Uterine Cancer
1939	42	F	Yakama	Lymphatic Cancer
1939	62	F	Yakama	Uterine Cancer
1940	33	M	Off Rez	Cancer of the Lung
1940	69	F	Off Rez	Uterine Cancer
1940	33	M	Off Rez	Lung Cancer
1941	79	F	Yakama	Stomach Cancer
1941	50	F	Yakama	Uterine Cancer
1941	79	F	Yakama	Stomach Breast/Bladder Cancers
1941	50	F	Yakama	Uterine Cancer
1942	83	F	Off Rez	Breast Cancer
1943	82	M	Off Rez	Bladder Cancer
1943	44	F	Off Rez	Breast Cancer
1943	82	M	Off Rez	Cancer of the Bladder
1943	44	F	Off Rez	Breast Cancer
1944	73	F	Yakama	Stomach Cancer
1944	40	M	Yakama	Leukemia
1945	72	F	Yakama	Uterine Cancer
1945	42	F	Off Rez	Cancer

Year	Age	Gender	Place	Explanation
1947	88	F	Off Rez	Breast Cancer
1947	50	F	Off Rez	Lung Cancer
1947	67	M	Yakama	Intestinal Cancer
1948	24	F	Off Rez	Lung Cancer
1948	48	F	Off Rez	Stomach Cancer
1949	69	F	Yakama	Uterine Cancer
1949	80	M	Yakama	Rectal Cancer
1949	—	F	Yakama	Cancer of the Liver
1950	68	F	Yakama	Uterine Cancer
1950	43	F	Off Rez	Breast Cancer
1950	36	M	Yakama	Brain Tumor
1951	74	M	Yakama	Cancer
1952	40	F	Yakama	Uterine Cancer
1952	64	F	Off Rez	Cancer of Gallbladder
1952	9	M	Off Rez	Leukemia
1953	70	F	Off Rez	Breast Cancer
1953	62	M	Yakama	Prostate Cancer
1953	74	F	Yakama	Pancreatic Cancer/Glycosuria
1953	39	F	Off Rez	Breast Cancer
1954	64	M	Yakama	Cancer Metastasis/Liver Lesion
1954	68	F	Off Rez	Carcinoma of Cervix/Metastasis
1954	81	F	Off Rez	Breast Carcinoma
1955	67	M	Yakama	Cancer of Stomach/Senility
1955	98	M	Off Rez	Stomach Carcinoma
1955	60	F	Yakama	Cancer of Uterus
1956	46	F	Yakama	Carcinoma of Cervix Uterine
1957	41	M	Yakama	Cancer of the Stomach
1957	58	F	Off Rez	Cancer of Uterus
1958	75	F	Yakama	Carcinoma Probably in Ovary
1959	85	M	Off Rez	Cancer of Prostate
1959	75	M	Off Rez	Carcinoma of Prostate
1959	94	F	Off Rez	Cancer of Tile Stomach
1960	60	F	Hospital	Malnutrition/Hemorrhage/Cancer
1961	63	F	Hospital	Carcinoma of Pancreas
1962	68	M	Off Rez	Respiratory
1962	67	M	Off Rez	Carcinoma
1962	74	M	Hospital	Adenocarcinoma
1962	3	M	Off Rez	Carcinoma of Liver/Metastasis
1962	70	M	Hospital	Anemia/Stomach Carcinoma
1963	47	F	Off Rez	Tumor/Edema
1964	47	F	Off Rez	Carcinoma of Cervix

Premature Birth

A BABY BORN BEFORE 37 WEEKS in the uterus is considered premature, and premature birth today is a common cause of death among infants. When Yakama women gave birth to a child prematurely, the internal organs of the infant may have suffered from underdevelopment or chromosomal abnormalities, putting the child at risk for diverse disorders. These problems could have been genetic or the result of the mother's condition, including kidney diseases, diabetes, high blood pressure, alcohol abuse, and connective tissue issues. Some mothers suffered from venereal disease, which contributed significantly to the premature birth. Today, medical scientists know that premature birth is more likely to occur among women who receive little or no prenatal care. Yakama women once received the expert prenatal help and knowledge of medicine women and midwives—people who helped other women for generations to prepare for birthing and postnatal care. Usually women within extended families helped one another with prenatal care, or specialists within the villages helped women prepare and give birth. However, the Plateau Indian War of 1855–1859 significantly disrupted families and prenatal care. And the reservation system continued the downward spiral of traditional medicine and a mother's help from midwives.

Over the years, midwives died and family units had fewer women to turn to for prenatal knowledge and help, at least until the 1910s, when the Office of Indian Affairs hired a few women to serve as matrons and offer "Well Baby Clinics," a program that attracted very few Yakama women at that time. During the late 19th and early 20th centuries, more women also relied on wage labor for their livelihoods. Working away from their homes in towns, on ranches, and at farms took men and women out of their homes and villages. Women lost access to traditional prenatal and postnatal care as a result of economic changes. The people continued to hunt, gather, and fish, but not to the extent they had prior to the mid-19th century. As a result of working for cash money, diets changed dramatically over the years and foods eaten, such as fry bread, pinto beans, and rice, did not provide the bodies of Plateau Indians the nutrition they had once enjoyed.

Yakama women sometimes gave birth to premature babies because of their own poor diets. According to the death certificates, only one child died as a result of malnutrition, a male baby born in a hospital in 1962. Still, the changing diets of Yakama mothers, resulting from the reservation system, likely caused the premature births of other babies, even though agents did not mention malnutrition. Today, malnutrition is a known cause of premature births, and this probably played a role historically in the deaths of Yakama infants. Furthermore, the lack of development of organs within the baby's body also led to premature births. In three cases, recording agents mentioned lung problems as a cause of premature birth. They also mentioned diarrhea and dehydration as causes for premature deaths. Another noted cause of premature births resulting in infant deaths proved to be syphilis, a cause that doomed the baby from the start. The health condition of other mothers also influenced the immune systems of their babies, and diseases contracted by mothers such as rubella, chickenpox, influenza, hepatitis, and other infections weakened both mothers and babies, sometimes causing premature births. Babies also died of birth defects brought on by many possible causes. However, the death certificates are not clear on most causes of the premature births, as they reported that the child died of "premature childbirth." Little is known about the exact causes for these deaths, but the factors mentioned above had to have had some influence on the shortened lives of babies born prematurely and the 41 stillbirths separately recorded in the death certificates. Officials at the reservation recorded over 100 premature and stillbirths, but it is likely that far more occurred and went unrecorded because families mourned the deaths of these little ones in their own way and buried them without reporting the death to white agents. These deaths were private affairs, not events that Indians wished to share with government agents.

Year	Age	Gender	Place	Explanation
1926	0	M	Yakama	Premature Birth
1926	0	F	Yakama	Hemorrhage/Premature
1926	0	M	Yakama	Premature Delivery
1926	0	F	Yakama	Premature Delivery
1926	0	M	Yakama	Premature Birth
1926	0	M	Yakama	Premature Birth
1927	0	F	Yakama	Immature Birth
1928	0	F	Yakama	Prematurity
1928	0	F	Yakama	Premature
1928	0	M	Yakama	Premature
1932	0	F	Yakama	Premature Childbirth
1936	0	M	Yakama	Premature
1936	0	M	Yakama	Premature
1936	0	M	Yakama	Premature Childbirth
1936	0	M	Yakama	Premature Childbirth
1936	0	M	Yakama	Premature Childbirth
1936	0	M	Yakama	Premature Childbirth
1937	0	M	Yakama	Premature Childbirth
1937	0	F	Yakama	Premature Childbirth
1937	0	F	Yakama	Premature Childbirth
1937	0	F	Yakama	Premature Childbirth
1937	0	M	Yakama	Premature Childbirth
1937	0	F	Yakama	Premature Childbirth
1939	0	F	Yakama	Premature Childbirth
1939	0	F	Yakama	Premature
1939	0	F	Off Rez	Premature
1940	0	M	Yakama	Premature
1940	0	F	Off Rez	Premature Childbirth/Syphilis
1940	0	M	Yakama	Atelectasis/Premature
1940	0	M	Yakama	Premature Childbirth/Syphilis
1940	0	M	Yakama	Premature Childbirth
1941	0	M	Yakama	Syphilis/Premature
1941	0	M	Off Rez	Premature
1941	0	M	Yakama	Premature Childbirth
1942	0	M	Yakama	Premature
1943	0	F	Yakama	Premature
1943	0	M	Yakama	Premature and Dehydration
1944	0	M	Yakama	Premature Childbirth
1944	0	M	Yakama	Premature Childbirth/Diarrhea
1945	0	F	Off Rez	Premature Childbirth

Year	Age	Gender	Place	Explanation
1946	0	M	Yakama	Premature Childbirth
1946	0	F	Yakama	Premature Childbirth
1947	0	M	Yakama	Premature Childbirth
1948	0	F	Off Rez	Premature Separation of Placenta
1948	0	F	Yakama	Premature Childbirth
1949	0	M	Yakama	Premature Childbirth
1949	0	M	Yakama	Premature Childbirth
1949	0	F	Yakama	Premature Childbirth
1953	0	M	Yakama	Premature Childbirth
1953	0	M	Yakama	Premature Childbirth
1954	0	F	Off Rez	Premature Labor
1955	0	F	Off Rez	Premature Childbirth
1956	0	M	Off Rez	Prematurity
1956	0	F	Off Rez	Prematurity
1957	0	M	Off Rez	Premature Development
1957	0	M	Off Rez	Prematurity
1958	0	F	Off Rez	Prematurity
1960	0	M	Off Rez	Atelectasis of Lungs/Premature
1962	0	M	Hospital	Malnutrition/Premature Childbirth
1962	0	M	Off Rez	Premature Childbirth
1962	0	F	Off Rez	Congenital Atelectasis/Premature
1963	0	M	Off Rez	Premature Childbirth
1964	0	M	Off Rez	Premature Childbirth

Old Age

Year	Age	Gender	Place	Explanation
1915	80	F	Yakama	Old Age
1915	85	M	Yakama	Old Age
1916	85	M	Yakama	Old Age
1918	83	F	Yakama	Old Age
1918	80	M	Yakama	Old Age
1918	74	M	Yakama	Old Age
1919	82	F	Yakama	Old Age
1925	67	M	Yakama	Senility
1925	65	F	Yakama	Senility
1925	85	M	Yakama	Senility
1925	70	F	Yakama	Senility
1925	72	F	Yakama	Senility
1925	69	M	Yakama	Senility
1925	83	M	Yakama	Senility
1925	78	F	Yakama	Senility
1925	75	F	Yakama	Senility
1925	72	F	Yakama	Senility
1925	92	F	Yakama	Senility
1925	78	M	Yakama	Senility
1925	80	M	Yakama	Senility
1925	85	M	Yakama	Senility
1926	73	F	Yakama	Senility
1926	82	M	Yakama	Senility

Year	Age	Gender	Place	Explanation
1926	99	M	Yakama	Old Age/Senility
1926	75	F	Yakama	Senility
1926	97	F	Yakama	Senility
1926	76	M	Yakama	Senility
1926	75	F	Yakama	Senility
1927	74	F	Yakama	Senility
1927	84	F	Yakama	Senility
1927	97	F	Off Rez	Senility
1927	83	F	Yakama	Senility
1927	99	F	Yakama	Old Age
1927	99	M	Yakama	Old Age
1927	73	F	Yakama	Old Age
1927	73	M	Yakama	Senility
1927	73	F	Yakama	Senility
1927	73	F	Yakama	Senility
1927	72	M	Yakama	Senility
1927	87	M	Yakama	Senility
1928	75	M	Yakama	Senility
1928	94	F	Yakama	Senility
1928	99	M	Yakama	Senility
1928	85	M	Yakama	Senility
1928	70	M	Yakama	Senility
1928	75	F	Yakama	Senility
1929	74	M	Yakama	Senility
1930	86	F	Yakama	Senility
1930	93	F	Yakama	Senility
1930	77	M	Yakama	Senility
1930	90	F	Off Rez	Senility
1931	65	M	Yakama	General Senility
1932	74	F	Yakama	Probably Senility
1932	80	F	Yakama	Probably Senility
1932	99	F	Yakama	Senility
1955	83	M	Yakama	Senility
1960	98	F	Hospital	Inanition/Debility/Senility

Stroke

When conditions within the body force blood flow to the brain to be cut off or disrupted, cells can die or become damaged from the lack of oxygen, and a stroke will likely occur. Furthermore, bleeding within or around the brain may cause a stroke. Medical scientists call these neurological problems "cerebrovascular disorders." When blood is cut off from part of the brain for brief periods of time, transient ischemic attacks or temporary malfunctioning of the brain takes place. In these cases, blood supplies return to the brain relatively quickly and brain cells are not destroyed. However, if a more serious cerebrovascular accident or stroke occurs, blood flow cannot feed the cells near or within the brain, and the person loses brain cells and tissues. Of course, this is far more serious, because of the death of brain cells. Insufficient oxygen to the brain creates permanent damage to the person who may have difficulty seeing, hearing, eating, moving their limbs, or thinking.

Year	Age	Gender	Place	Explanation
1925	62	M	Yakama	Cerebral Embolism
1925	62	M	Yakama	Cerebral Embolism
1927	60	F	Yakama	Cerebral Hemorrhage
1928	74	F	Off Rez	Cerebral Hemorrhage
1931	76	F	Yakama	Apoplexy
1931	76	F	Yakama	Cerebral Hemorrhage
1934	75	F	Yakama	Cerebral Hemorrhage
1934	75	F	Yakama	Cerebral Hemorrhage
1937	94	F	Off Rez	Cerebral Hemorrhage
1937	94	M	Yakama	Cerebral Hemorrhage
1939	60	M	Yakama	Cerebral Hemorrhage/ Arteriosclerosis
1939	60	M	Off Rez	Cerebral Hemorrhage/ Arteriosclerosis
1941	68	M	Off Rez	Cerebral Hemorrhage
1941	83	F	Off Rez	Cerebral Hemorrhage/ Arteriosclerosis
1941	—	M	Yakama	Cerebral Hemorrhage
1943	74	F	Yakama	Cerebral Hemorrhage/ Hypertension
1943	74	F	Yakama	Cerebral Hemorrhage
1944	76	F	Yakama	Cerebral Hemorrhage
1944	64	F	Off Rez	Cerebral Hemorrhage
1945	55	F	Off Rez	Cerebral Hemorrhage
1945	0	M	Yakama	Birth Injury/Cerebral Hemorrhage
1947	67	M	Yakama	Cerebral Accident (Stroke)
1948	79	M	Off Rez	Cerebral Hemorrhage
1950	85	F	Yakama	Stroke/Cardiac Degeneration
1951	60	F	Yakama	Cerebral Hemorrhage
1952	85	M	Off Rez	Stroke/Heart Disease
1952	86	M	Yakama	Cerebral Hemorrhage
1953	45	F	Yakama	Cerebral Hemorrhage
1954	56	F	Off Rez	Cerebral Hemorrhage
1954	70	M	Off Rez	Cerebral Hemorrhage
1955	68	M	Off Rez	Cerebral Hemorrhage
1955	75	M	Off Rez	Cerebral Hemorrhage
1956	67	M	Off Rez	Cerebral Vascular Accident
1956	70	M	Off Rez	Cerebral Thrombosis/Diabetes
1957	72	F	Off Rez	Cerebral Vascular Accident
1957	54	F	Off Rez	Cerebral Hemorrhage

Year	Age	Gender	Place	Explanation
1957	72	F	Off Rez	Cerebral Vascular Accident
1957	81	F	Off Rez	Cerebral Vascular Accident
1958	1	M	Off Rez	Cerebral Vascular Accident
1958	69	M	Off Rez	Cerebral Vascular Accident
1959	79	F	Yakama	Cerebral Vascular Accident
1959	44	F	Off Rez	Cerebral Vascular Accident
1959	47	M	Off Rez	Cerebral Vascular Accident
1959	51	M	Off Rez	Cerebral Vascular Accident
1961	87	F	Off Rez	Cerebral Vascular Accident

Alcoholism

Year	Age	Gender	Place	Explanation
1926	62	M	Yakama	Auto Accident/Drunk Driving
1926	76	M	Yakama	Poisoned by Wood Alcohol
1929	33	M	Yakama	Acute Alcoholism
1929	35	M	Yakama	Acute Alcoholism
1932	31	M	Yakama	Acute Alcoholism
1932	31	M	Off Rez	Acute Alcoholism
1933	55	F	Yakama	Alcohol Poisoning
1933	55	F	Yakama	Poisoning by Denatured Alcohol
1934	63	F	Yakama	Acute Alcoholism
1934	63	F	Yakama	Acute Alcoholism
1936	32	M	Yakama	Wood Alcohol Poisoning
1936	62	F	Off Rez	Alcoholism
1936	24	F	Off Rez	Alcoholism
1936	74	M	Yakama	Wood Alcohol Poison/Husband
1936	70	F	Yakama	Wood Alcohol Poisoning/Wife
1936	28	F	Off Rez	Wood Alcohol Poisoning
1936	28	F	Off Rez	Wood Alcohol Poisoning
1936	32	M	Yakama	Wood Alcohol Poisoning
1936	28	F	Off Rez	Wood Alcohol Poisoning
1936	76	F	Off Rez	Wood Alcohol Poisoning
1936	74	M	Yakama	Wood Alcohol Poisoning
1936	24	F	Yakama	Wood Alcohol Poisoning
1938	41	M	Yakama	Auto Accident Due to Alcohol

Year	Age	Gender	Place	Explanation
1939	50	M	Yakama	Alcoholism
1939	70	M	Yakama	Alcoholism
1939	70	M	Yakama	Alcoholism
1939	50	M	Yakama	Alcoholism
1941	48	F	Off Rez	Alcohol
1943	81	M	Yakama	Alcohol
1943	86	M	Yakama	Alcohol
1949	29	M	Yakama	Alcohol
1950	38	M	Off Rez	Alcohol
1950	43	M	Yakama	Alcohol
1952	36	M	Yakama	Nephritis/Alcoholism
1954	40	F	Off Rez	Acute Alcoholism/Drinking
1956	38	M	Yakama	Hepatic Cirrhosis/Alcoholism
1957	46	F	Off Rez	Acute Alcoholism
1958	50	M	Yakama	Hepatic Coma/Alcoholism
1958	42	F	Off Rez	Gastrointestinal Hemorrhage
1959	48	M	Yakama	Car Overturned/Alcoholism
1960	28	F	Off Rez	Methanol Intoxication/Alcoholism
1961	47	M	Yakama	Cirrhosis of Liver/Alcoholism
1961	42	F	Off Rez	Liver Failure/Cirrhosis/Alcohol
1961	46	M	Yakama	Signs of Acute Alcoholism
1962	32	F	Off Rez	Cirrhosis/Alcoholism
1962	61	M	Off Rez	Diabetic Acidosis/Alcoholism
1962	44	F	Off Rez	Liver Failure/Alcoholism
1962	37	F	Hospital	Liver Failure/Alcoholism
1963	39	F	Off Rez	Hepatic Failure/Alcoholic
1964	45	F	Off Rez	Liver Failure/Alcoholism
1964	53	M	Off Rez	Liver Failure/Alcoholism

Natural Causes

Year	Age	Gender	Place	Explanation
1929	77	M	Yakama	Natural Causes
1931	90	M	Yakama	Natural Causes
1931	60	F	Yakama	Natural Causes
1932	74	F	Yakama	Natural Causes
1932	76	F	Yakama	Natural Causes
1932	99	F	Yakama	Natural Causes
1940	94	M	Yakama	Natural Causes
1940	95	F	Yakama	Natural Causes
1940	91	M	Yakama	Natural Causes
1940	95	F	Off Rez	Natural Causes
1940	85	F	Off Rez	Natural Causes
1941	89	F	Yakama	Natural Causes
1941	—	M	Yakama	Anemia/Natural Causes
1942	99	M	Off Rez	Natural Causes
1943	70	F	Yakama	Natural Causes
1943	94	M	Off Rez	Natural Causes
1943	70	F	Yakama	Natural Causes
1943	83	M	Yakama	Natural Causes
1943	99	M	Yakama	Natural Causes
1944	80	M	Yakama	Natural Causes
1944	69	F	Yakama	Carbuncle/Natural Causes
1945	79	F	Off Rez	Natural Causes
1945	89	F	Yakama	Natural Causes

Year	Age	Gender	Place	Explanation
1945	7	F	Off Rez	Natural Causes
1946	84	F	Off Rez	Natural Causes
1946	90	F	Off Rez	Natural Causes
1947	76	F	Off Rez	Natural Causes
1947	75	M	Yakama	Natural Causes
1947	99	F	Yakama	Natural Causes
1948	98	M	Yakama	Natural Causes
1948	99	M	Yakama	Natural Causes
1948	99	F	Yakama	Natural Causes
1948	83	F	Off Rez	Natural Causes
1948	86	F	Yakama	Natural Causes
1949	99	F	Yakama	Natural Causes
1950	82	M	Yakama	Natural Causes
1951	99	F	Yakama	Natural Causes
1951	96	F	Yakama	Natural Causes
1951	99	M	Off Rez	Natural Causes

Kidney

Year	Age	Gender	Place	Explanation
1924	48	M	Yakama	Kidney Trouble
1931	26	M	Yakama	Nephritis
1931	36	M	Yakama	Acute Nephritis
1932	68	F	Yakama	Diabetes
1932	52	M	Yakama	Nephritis
1932	98	F	Yakama	Nephritis
1932	98	F	Yakama	Chronic Nephritis
1932	52	M	Yakama	Chronic Nephritis
1933	48	F	Off Rez	Diabetes
1934	70	F	Yakama	Nephritis/Influenza
1935	78	M	Yakama	Arthritis/Nephritis/Uremia
1937	70	F	Yakama	Nephritis
1939	63	F	Yakama	Nephritis/Edema/Renal Failure
1939	63	F	Yakama	Nephritis with Edema/Renal Failure
1940	65	M	Off Rez	Nephritis/Uremia
1940	65	M	Off Rez	Nephritis
1941	71	M	Off Rez	Diabetes
1941	71	M	Off Rez	Diabetes
1943	74	M	Yakama	Pylonephritis/Prostate
1943	63	M	Yakama	Diabetes
1943	—	M	Yakama	Diabetes
1945	52	M	Off Rez	Nephritis and Uremia
1945	31	F	Off Rez	Nephritis

Year	Age	Gender	Place	Explanation
1952	43	F	Off Rez	Nephritis/Tuberculosis/Cancer
1955	0	M	Off Rez	Toxic Nephritis/Myocarditis
1957	34	F	Off Rez	Toxic Hepatitis
1958	51	M	Yakama	Uremia/Chronic Nephritis
1959	45	M	Off Rez	Diabetes/Acute Pancreatitis
1960	64	F	Off Rez	Diabetes Mellitis
1961	93	F	Off Rez	Uremia Coma/Pyelonephritis
1961	45	M	Off Rez	Acidosis/Diabetes
1963	33	F	Off Rez	Arrhythmia/Uremia/Pylonephritis
1964	66	M	Off Rez	Perirenal Abscess

Hemorrhage

Year	Age	Gender	Place	Explanation
1931	16	F	Yakama	Typhoid Ulcer with Hemorrhage
1934	36	F	Off Rez	Jaundice/Internal Hemorrhage
1938	0	M	Yakama	Intestinal Hemorrhaging
1938	0	M	Yakama	Umbilical Hemorrhage at Birth
1938	78	M	Yakama	Hemorrhage from Ulcer
1939	0	F	Yakama	Newborn Hemorrhagic Disease
1939	0	F	Yakama	Newborn Hemorrhagic Disease
1940	0	M	Off Rez	Hemorrhagic Disease/Premature
1946	77	M	Yakama	Stomach Hemorrhage/Heart Disease
1949	75	F	Off Rez	Hemorrhage
1953	85	F	Off Rez	Gastrointestinal Hemorrhage
1954	82	M	Off Rez	Hemorrhage/Stomach Cancer
1954	51	M	Yakama	Ulcer of Stomach
1954	22	M	Off Rez	Internal Hemorrhage
1955	0	M	Off Rez	Newborn Hemorrhagic Disease
1955	23	F	Off Rez	Hemorrhage and Shock
1955	69	M	Off Rez	Ulcers/Hemorrhage
1957	69	M	Off Rez	Cranial Hemorrhage
1958	70	F	Off Rez	Narcosis of Liver/Hemorrhage
1959	65	M	Off Rez	Gastrointestinal Hemorrhage
1959	86	—	Off Rez	Gastrointestinal Hemorrhage
1959	66	M	Off Rez	Gastrointestinal Hemorrhage

Year	Age	Gender	Place	Explanation
1960	40	M	Off Rez	Gastrointestinal Hemorrhage
1961	99	F	Off Rez	Rectal Hemorrhage
1961	48	F	Off Rez	Gastrointestinal Hemorrhage
1962	54	M	Off Rez	Gastrointestinal Hemorrhage
1963	0	M	Off Rez	Hemorrhage

Whooping Cough

Year	Age	Gender	Place	Explanation
1918	5	F	Yakama	Whooping Cough
1918	3	F	Yakama	Whooping Cough
1925	0	M	Yakama	Whooping Cough
1925	0	F	Yakama	Whooping Cough
1925	1	M	Yakama	Whooping Cough
1925	2	M	Yakama	Whooping Cough
1925	1	F	Yakama	Whooping Cough
1925	0	F	Off Rez	Whooping Cough
1925	1	M	Yakama	Whooping Cough
1926	0	F	Yakama	Whooping Cough
1926	1	F	Yakama	Whooping Cough
1928	4	M	Off Rez	Whooping Cough
1930	2	M	Yakama	Whooping Cough
1930	2	M	Yakama	Whooping Cough
1932	1	M	Yakama	Whooping Cough
1932	1	M	Yakama	Whooping Cough
1941	2	F	Off Rez	Whooping Cough
1946	1	F	Yakama	Whooping Cough
1950	0	M	Yakama	Whooping Cough
1954	11	F	Yakama	Whooping Cough

Stillborn

Year	Age	Gender	Place	Explanation
1931	0	M	Yakama	Stillborn
1931	0	F	Yakama	Slow Delivery of Head/Podalic
1931	0	F	Yakama	Stillborn
1932	0	M	Yakama	Stillborn/Premature Birth
1938	0	M	Yakama	Hemorrhaging after Birth
1942	0	F	Yakama	Born Dead
1945	0	M	Yakama	Birth Injury
1945	0	F	Yakama	Birth Injury
1958	0	F	Off Rez	Stillbirth
1960	0	M	Off Rez	Stillbirth
1960	0	F	Off Rez	Stillbirth/Twisted Cord
1960	0	M	Hospital	Stillbirth/Prematurity
1961	0	F	Off Rez	Stillbirth
1961	0	M	Off Rez	Stillbirth
1962	0	F	Off Rez	Stillbirth
1963	0	M	Off Rez	Stillbirth
1963	0	F	Off Rez	Stillbirth
1964	0	M	Hospital	Stillbirth
1964	0	M	Off Rez	Stillbirth/Breech Delivery

Venereal Disease

Year	Age	Gender	Place	Explanation
1938	0	F	Yakama	Gonorrheal Opthalmia
1939	0	M	Yakama	Congenital Syphilis
1939	2	M	Yakama	Syphilis
1939	0	M	Yakama	Syphilis
1940	0	M	Yakama	Syphilis
1940	0	M	Off Rez	Syphilis/Premature
1940	0	M	Yakama	Syphilis
1940	0	M	Off Rez	Syphilis/Premature
1941	0	F	Yakama	Syphilis
1941	24	F	Off Rez	Syphilis
1941	24	F	Off Rez	Syphilis
1942	66	M	Off Rez	Syphilis
1942	0	F	Yakama	Syphilis
1942	0	F	Yakama	Syphilis
1944	1	M	Yakama	Syphilis
1944	0	M	Yakama	Convulsion Due to Congenital Syphilis
1944	0	M	Yakama	Syphilis
1944	0	M	Yakama	Syphilis
1954	68	M	Off Rez	Syphilitic Aortitis

Blood Poisoning

Year	Age	Gender	Place	Explanation
1925	57	M	Yakama	Blood Poisoning
1927	63	F	Yakama	Septicemia
1928	52	M	Yakama	Septicemia
1928	63	F	Yakama	Septicemia
1932	44	M	Off Rez	Septicemia Due to Prostate
1933	72	F	Off Rez	Blood Poisoning
1934	26	M	Off Rez	Septicemia/Abscessed Tonsil
1937	12	M	Yakama	Septicemia
1937	12	M	Off Rez	Septicemia Following Injury
1939	15	F	Yakama	Blood Poisoning
1939	15	F	Yakama	Blood Poisoning
1940	0	M	Yakama	Septicemia from Childbirth
1940	0	M	Yakama	Septicemia Following Childbirth
1943	22	F	Off Rez	Gangrene/Septicemia
1944	0	M	Yakama	Septicemia, Thyroid or Encephalic
1944	80	F	Yakama	Septicemia from Nail Wound
1944	80	F	Yakama	Septicemia
1945	42	F	Off Rez	Septicemia from Miscarriage

Exposure

Year	Age	Gender	Place	Explanation
1927	0	M	Yakama	Exposure
1927	0	F	Yakama	Exposure
1927	0	M	Yakama	Exposure
1928	0	F	Yakama	Exposure
1928	78	M	Off Rez	Exposure/Body Found in Field
1933	75	M	Yakama	Alcoholism and Exposure
1935	80	M	Yakama	Exposure/Fell in Creek
1942	85	F	Yakama	Heat Stroke
1942	46	M	Yakama	Heat Stroke while Intoxicated
1942	35	M	Yakama	Heat Stroke
1942	36	M	Yakama	Heat Stroke
1950	70	F	Yakama	Exposure after Fall
1956	72	M	Yakama	Signs of Alcoholism/Exposure
1960	49	M	Hospital	Exhaustion/Exposure
1962	42	M	Hospital	Hypothermia/Exposure
1964	77	F	Off Rez	Exposure and Alcoholism

Surgical Complications

Year	Age	Gender	Place	Explanation
1931	6	M	Yakama	Respiratory Paralysis during Surgery
1931	6	M	Yakama	Accidentally Taking Ether
1932	46	M	Off Rez	Cholecystitis/Mild Surgical Shock
1932	57	F	Off Rez	Heart Stoppage in Surgery
1932	20	M	Yakama	Infection following Appendicitis
1932	48	F	Off Rez	Anuria from Hysterectomy
1932	20	M	Yakama	Pulmonary Abscess Post-Op
1937	31	F	Off Rez	Surgical Shock/Hysterectomy
1937	31	M	Off Rez	Surgical Shock
1938	12	M	Yakama	Hemorrhage after Tonsillectomy
1942	75	M	Off Rez	Surgical Shock/Cancer
1943	11	M	Off Rez	Surgical Shock
1948	24	F	Off Rez	Respiratory and Heart Failure
1953	69	M	Off Rez	Pulmonary Embolus after Surgery
1953	36	M	Off Rez	Post-Operative Pulmonary Embolus

Bronchitis

Year	Age	Gender	Place	Explanation
1929	54	F	Yakama	Bronchitis
1929	54	F	Off Rez	Bronchiectasis
1938	46	F	Yakama	Bronchitis/Asthma
1939	22	F	Off Rez	Respiratory Failure
1939	22	F	Off Rez	Respiratory Failure/Dysentery
1946	4	F	Yakama	Respiratory Failure
1948	0	F	Off Rez	Bronchitis/Hypertension
1954	0	F	Off Rez	Dehydration/Respiratory Infection
1954	0	F	Yakama	Respiratory Infection/Rickets
1954	0	M	Off Rez	Acute Bronchitis
1955	0	M	Yakama	Laryngs-Traches/Bronchitis
1955	77	M	Yakama	Signs of Lung Complication
1963	0	M	Hospital	Tracheobronchitis
1964	0	M	Off Rez	Respiratory Arrest

Paralysis

Year	Age	Gender	Place	Explanation
1924	41	M	Yakama	Paralysis
1924	27	F	Yakama	Paralysis
1927	40	M	Yakama	Dementia/Paralysis
1927	25	F	Off Rez	Paralysis
1927	18	M	Yakama	Paralysis
1928	56	M	Yakama	Paralysis
1928	56	M	Yakama	Paralyzed/Grew Weaker
1931	6	M	Yakama	Paralyzed
1931	73	M	Yakama	Paralysis
1934	16	M	Off Rez	Probable Infantile Paralysis
1934	0	F	Yakama	Infantile Paralysis
1934	0	F	Yakama	Infantile Paralysis
1934	16	M	Off Rez	Infantile Paralysis

Liver Disorders

Year	Age	Gender	Place	Explanation
1925	51	M	Yakama	Liver/Stomach Trouble
1928	57	F	Off Rez	Jaundice
1949	32	M	Yakama	Rupture of Liver/Internal Hemorrhage
1957	11	F	Off Rez	Hepatic Failure/Cirrhosis
1959	51	F	Off Rez	Hepatic Failure
1959	58	M	Off Rez	Hepatic Coma/Diabetes
1961	48	F	Off Rez	Cirrhosis Of Liver
1963	68	F	Off Rez	Hepatic Cirrhosis/Bile Duct
1963	29	F	Off Rez	Cirrhosis of Liver
1964	53	F	Off Rez	Hepatic Coma/Hepatitis
1964	60	M	Off Rez	Renal Failure/Hepatic Cirrhosis
1964	32	F	Hospital	Hepatitis Fatty Degeneration

Typhoid

Year	Age	Gender	Place	Explanation
1911	5	M	Yakama	Typhoid/Pneumonia
1911	38	F	Yakama	Typhoid
1926	11	M	Yakama	Typhoid/Fever
1928	28	M	Yakama	Typhoid/Fever
1931	17	M	Yakama	Typhoid
1931	17	M	Yakama	Typhoid Fever
1932	16	M	Yakama	Typhoid/Ulcer/Mild Hemorrhage
1939	52	F	Yakama	Typhoid
1940	7	F	Off Rez	Typhoid
1940	7	F	Off Rez	Typhoid
1941	0	F	Off Rez	Typhoid
1946	53	M	Off Rez	Typhoid Fever

Measles

Year	Age	Gender	Place	Explanation
1924	0	F	Yakama	Measles and Bad Cold
1924	0	F	Yakama	Measles and Bad Cold
1925	1	M	Yakama	Measles
1928	5	F	Off Rez	Measles
1931	0	M	Yakama	Measles and Bronchopneumonia
1931	14	F	Yakama	Bronchopneumonia following Measles
1931	14	M	Yakama	Measles
1939	1	M	Yakama	Measles/Pneumonia
1940	0	M	Yakama	Measles/Pneumonia
1962	0	F	Off Rez	Measles

Suffocation

Year	Age	Gender	Place	Explanation
1940	0	M	Yakama	Asphyxiation from Wrapping
1940	0	M	Off Rez	Suffocation
1941	0	F	Off Rez	Accidental Asphyxia
1943	0	M	Off Rez	Suffocation
1943	0	M	Yakama	Suffocation
1946	0	M	Off Rez	Suffocation
1960	0	M	Hospital	Asphyxia, Malnutrition, Diarrhea

Encephalitis

Year	Age	Gender	Place	Explanation
1926	36	M	Yakama	Encephalitis
1926	36	M	Yakama	Encephalitis
1930	56	M	Yakama	Encephalitis
1931	20	F	Yakama	Meningoencephalitis
1933	12	M	Off Rez	Encephalitis
1939	0	M	Yakama	Encephalitis
1952	1	M	Off Rez	Meningoencephalitis

Appendicitis

Year	Age	Gender	Place	Explanation
1925	17	F	Yakama	Appendicitis
1927	2	F	Yakama	Appendicitis
1927	2	F	Yakama	Appendicitis
1928	7	F	Off Rez	Ruptured Appendix
1930	6	M	Yakama	Acute Appendicitis
1930	6	M	Yakama	Appendicitis
1946	55	F	Yakama	Appendicitis/Peritonitis

Bibliography

Manuscript Collections

Click Relander Collection. Yakima Valley Regional Library, Yakima, Washington.

Dean and Geraldine Guie Collection. Mourning Dove's autobiographical manuscript and traditional stories. Private collection, Yakima, Washington.

Death Certificates, Agency Letterbooks, Birth Records. Yakima Agency Records. National Archives, Pacific Northwest, Seattle, Washington.

George Birkby, Jones Jim, Kamiakin, Patrick Nightwalker, Peone Interviews; Bartlett, Scheuerman, and Seeman Manuscripts; Palouse Indian Calendar; Kamiakin Geneaology. Department of Native American Studies, University of California, Riverside, California.

Granville O. Haller Collection. Bancroft Library, University of California, Berkeley.

Lucullus Virgil McWhorter Collection. Manuscripts, Archives, and Special Collections. Washington State University, Pullman, Washington.

Records of the Bureau of Indian Affairs. War Department, State Department, Indian Claims Commission, National Archives, Washington, D.C.

William Compton Brown Collection. Manuscripts Archives and Special Collections. Washington State University, Pullman, Washington.

World Population Data Sheet. Population Reference Bureau, Inc., Washington, D.C., 1983.

Original Sources

Alien, Paul. *History of the Expedition under the Command of Captains Lewis and Clark.* London: Longman, Hurst, Rees, Orme, and Brown, 1814.

Annual Reports of the Commissioners of Indian Affairs. Washington, D.C.: Government Printing Office.

Ault, Nelson A., ed. *The Papers of Lucullus Virgil McWhorter.* Pullman: Washington State College, 1959.

Benson, Todd. "Race, Health, and Power: The Federal Government and American Indian Health, 1909–1965." PhD diss., Stanford University, 1993.

Bischoff, William N. "The Yakima Indian War: 1855–1856." PhD diss., Loyola University of Chicago, 1950.

Blanchet, Francis Norbert. *Historical Sketches of the Catholic Church of Oregon.* Portland: Catholic Sentinel, 1878.

Boyd, Robert T. "The Introduction of Infectious Diseases among the Indians of the Pacific Northwest, 1774–1874." PhD diss., University of Washington, 1985.

Brown, William Compton. *The Indian Side of the Story.* Spokane: C. W. Hill Printing Company, 1961.

Bureau of Indian Affairs. *Report on the Source, Nature and Extent of Fishing, Hunting and Miscellaneous Related Rights of Certain Tribes in Oregon and Washington.* Los Angeles: Office of Indian Affairs, Division of Forestry and Grazing, 1942.

Chalfant, Stewart. *Ethno-historical Report on Aboriginal Land Occupancy and Utilization by the Palus Indians.* Defense Exhibit 69, United States Indian Claims Commission, National Archives, Record Group 279.

Chittenden, H. M., and A. T. Richardson, eds. *Life, Letters and Travels of Father Pierre-Jean DeSmet, S. J., 1801–1873: Missionary Labors and Adventures among the Wild Tribes of the North American Indians, Embracing Minute Descriptions of their Manners, Customs, Modes of Warfare and Torture.* 4 volumes. New York: Francis P. Harper, 1905.

Clayman, Charles B., ed. *The American Medical Association Encyclopedia of Medicine.* New York: Random House, 1989.

Coan, Charles F. "Federal Indian Policy in the Pacific Northwest, 1849–1870." PhD diss., University of California, 1920.

Cox, Ross. *Adventures on the Columbia River.* 2 volumes. London: H. Colburn and R. Bentley, 1831. Reprinted in 1957 by University of Oklahoma Press as *The Columbia River.*

Curtis, Edward S. *Indian Days of the Long Ago.* New York: World Book Company, 1915.

———. *The North American Indians.* Norwood, Mass.: Plimpton Press, 1911.

DeSmet, Pierre-Jean. *Oregon Missions and Travels over the Rocky Mountains in 1845–46.* New York: Edward Dunigan, 1847.

———. *Origin, Progress and Prospects of the Catholic Mission to the Rocky Mountains.* Philadelphia: M. Fithian, 1843.

Documents Relating to Negotiations of Ratified and Unratified Treaties. National Archives, Record Group 75. Microfilm T 494, Reel 5.

"Doty's Journal of Operations." Documents Relating to Negotiations of Ratified and Unratified Treaties. National Archives, Record Group 75. Microfilm T494. Reel 5.

DuBois, Cora. *The Feather Cult of the Middle Columbia.* General Series in Anthropology 7. Menasha, Wis.: George Banta Publishing Company, 1938.

Elliott, T. C., ed. "David Thompson's Journeys in the Spokane Country." *Washington Historical Quarterly* 8 (1917): 183–87, 261–64; 9 (1918): 11–16, 103–6, 169–73, 284–87; 10 (1919): 17–20.

———. "Journal of David Thompson." *Oregon Historical Quarterly* 15 (1914): 39–63, 104–25.

Franchere, Gabriel. *Narrative of a Voyage to the Northwest Coast of America in the Years 1811, 1812, 1813, and 1814, Or the First American Settlement on the Pacific.* New York: Redfield, 1854.

Gibbs, George. "Tribes of Western Washington and Northwestern Oregon Published with Extensive Vocabularies." In *Tribes of the Extreme Northwest, Contributions to North American Ethnology, 1*, for *United States Geographical and Geological Survey of the Rocky Mountain Region*, ed. W. H. Dall, 163–361. J. W. Powell, Director. Washington, D.C.: Bureau of American Ethnology, 1877.

Gibbs, George, et al. "Report on the Indian Tribes of the Territory of Washington." *Secretary of War Reports of Explorations 1* (1854): 400–449: see *House Executive Document 91*, 33rd Cong. 1st Sess., and reprinted in 1972 by Ye Galleon Press, Fairfield, Washington.

Gilbert, Frank T. *Historic Sketches of Walla Walla, Whitman, Columbia and Garfield Counties, Washington Territory.* Portland, Oregon: A. G. Walling Co., 1882.

Haller, Granville O. "Kamiakin—In History: Memoir of the War, in the Yakima Valley, 1855–1856." Manuscript A128, Bancroft Library, University of California, Berkeley.

Holy Bible. New York: Oxford University Press, 1973.

Howard, Oliver O. *My Life and Experiences among Our Hostile Indians: A Report of Personal Observations, Adventures, and Campaigns among the Indians of the Great West, with Some Account of Their Life, Habits, Traits, Religion, Ceremonies, Dress, Savage Instincts, and Customs in Peace and War.* Hartford: A. D. Worthington and Co., 1907.

———. *Nez Perce Joseph.* Boston: Lee and Sheperd, 1881.

Hunter, George. *Reminiscences of an Old Timer.* San Francisco: H. S. Crocker and Co., 1887.

Indian Claims Commission. "Evidence in Support of Proposed Findings of Fact of Petitioners in Docket Number 222 on Issues of Liability." United States Claims Commission. National Archives, Record Group 279.

———. "Testimony of Verne L. Ray." United States Claims Commission. National Archives, Record Group 279.

Indian Claims Commission Decisions. Volume 7, Part B and Volume 12, Part A. Boulder, Colo.: Native American Rights Fund, n.d.

Indian Health Service. *California Area 1993 Profile.* Sacramento: California Area Office, Indian Health Service, 1994.

———. *Regional Differences in Indian Health.* Washington, D.C.: United States Department of Health, Indian Health Service, 1993.

———. *Trends in Indian Health, 1991.* Washington, D.C.: United States Department of Health and Human Services, 1991.

Jim, Mary. "A Palouse Indian Speaks." *Bunchgrass Historian* 8 (1980): 20–23.

Johansen, Dorothy C., ed. *Robert Newell's Memoranda.* Portland: Champoeg Press, 1959.

Kappler, Charles J. *Indian Affairs, Laws and Treaties.* 2 volumes. Washington, D.C.: Government Printing Office, 1940.

Keeley, Patrick. "Nutrient Composition of Selected Important Plant Foods of the Precontact Diet of the Northwestern Native American Peoples." Master's thesis, University of Washington, 1980.

Kip, Lawrence. *Army Life on the Pacific: A Journal of the Expedition against the Northern Indians, the Tribes of the Coeur d'Alenes, Spokanes, and Pelouzes, in the Summer of 1858.* New York: Redfield Publishing Co., 1859.

Koenig, Margaret W. *Tuberculosis among the Nebraska Winnebago: A Social Study on an Indian Reservation.* Lincoln: Nebraska State Historical Society, 1921.

Kuykendall, G. B. *Spirit Beliefs.* Unpublished manuscript. Relander Collection, Yakima Valley Regional Library, Yakima, Washington.

Langone, Stephen A. "A Statistical Profile of the Indian: The Lack of Numbers." *United States Congress, Joint Economic Committee, Toward Economic Development for Native American Communities.* Vol. 2. Washington D.C.: Government Printing Office, 1969.

Manual X: Indirect Techniques for Demographic Estimations. Population Studies, Number 81, United Nations. New York: Department of International Economic and Social Affairs, 1983.

Manypenny, George W. *Our Indian Wards.* New York: Da Capo Press, Inc., 1972.

Masterson, James R. "The Records of the Washington Superintendency of Indian Affairs, 1853–1874." *Pacific Northwest Quarterly* 37 (1946): 31–41.

McWhorter, Luceullus Virgil. *Hear Me, My Chiefs!* Caldwell, Idaho: Caxton Printers, Ltd., 1952.

———. *Tragedy of the Whak-Shum; Prelude to the Yakima Indian War, 1855–56: The Killing of Major Andrew J. Bolon.* Fairfield, Wash.: Ye Galleon Press, 1958.

Meriam, Lewis. *The Problem of Indian Administration.* New York: Johnson Reprint Corporation, 1971.

Merk, Frederick, ed. *Fur Trade and Empire: George Simpson's Journal, 1824–1825.* Cambridge, Mass.: Belknap Press, 1968.

Mermel, T. W., ed. and comp. *Register of Dams in the United States: Completed, Under Construction and Proposed.* New York: McGraw Hill, 1958.

Merrit, Edgar B. "Health Conditions Among Indians." *Redman* (1914): 347–50.

Mooney, James. "The Ghost Dance Religion and the Sioux Outbreak of 1890." *Fourteenth Annual Report to the Bureau of American Ethnology.* Washington, D.C.: Government Printing Office, 1892–1893.

Moran, John, Evelyn Broncheau, Corky Covington, Pam Garza, Sharon John, Jim Horst, Linda Kafford, Karen Schmidt, and Jim Sutherland (Yakima Indian Health Center Morbidity and Mortality Committee). "1991 Mortality Report." Toppenish, Wash.: Yakima Indian Health Center, Yakima Nation, 1992.

Morton, Arthur S., ed. "The North West Company's Columbia Enterprise and David Thompson." *Canadian Historical Review* 17 (1936): 266–88; 18 (1937): 156–62.

Moulton, Gary, ed. *Journals of Lewis and Clark.* 7 volumes. Lincoln: University of Nebraska Press, 1983–1990.

Mullan, John. *Report on the Construction of a Military Road from Fort Walla Walla to Fort Benton.* Washington, D.C.: Government Printing Office, 1863.

———. "Report on the Indian Tribes in the Eastern Portion of Washington Territory, 1853." *Secretary of War, Reports of Explorations 1*, 437–41. Washington, D.C.: Government Printing Office, 1853.
———. "Topographical Memoir and Map of Colonel Wright's Late Campaign against the Indians of Oregon and Washington Territories." *Senate Executive Document*, 35th Congress, 2nd Session, No. 32, SS 984.
Official Register of the United States, 1883. Washington, D.C.: Government Printing Office, 1889.
Official Register of the United States, 1889. Washington, D.C.: Government Printing Office, 1891.
Official Register of the United States, 1893. Washington, D.C.: Government Printing Office, 1893.
Official Register of the United States, 1895. Washington, D.C.: Government Printing Office, 1895.
Official Register of the United States, 1897. Washington, D.C.: Government Printing Office, 1897.
Pambrun, Andrew D. *Sixty Years on the Frontier in the Pacific Northwest*. Ed. Edward J. Kowrach. Fairfield, Wash.: Ye Galleon Press, 1978.
Putney, Diane T. "Fighting the Scourge: American Indian Morbidity and Federal Policy, 1897–1930." PhD diss., Marquette University, 1980.
Puyallup Tribe v. Department of Game. 391 U.S. 392 (1968).
Quaife, Milo Milton. *Adventures of the First Settlers on the Oregon or Columbia River*. Chicago: Lakeside Press, 1923.
Ray, Verne F. "Economic Use of the Tribal Territory of the Yakima." United States Indian Claims Commission, Dockets 47 and 47A, National Archives, Record Group 279.
Relander, Click. *Sophie Williams' Interview in Colville and Palouse Notes*. Unpublished manuscript. Relander Collection. Yakima Valley Regional Library, Yakima, Washington.
Ross, Alexander. *Adventures of the First Settlers on the Oregon or Columbia River: Being a Narrative of the Expedition Fitted Out by John Jacob Astor to Establish the "Pacific Fur Company"; With an Account of Some Indian Tribes on the Coast of the Pacific*. London: Smith, Elder and Company, 1849.
———. *The Fur Hunters of the Far West; A Narrative of Adventures in the Oregon and Rocky Mountains*. Norman: University of Oklahoma Press, 1956.
Schmeckebier, Laurence F. *The Office of Indian Affairs: Its History, Activities, and Organization*. Institute for Government Research, Service Monographs of the United States, No. 48. Baltimore: Johns Hopkins Press, 1927.
Schoolcraft, Henry Rowe. *Historical and Statistical Information Respecting the History, Conditions, and Prospects of the Indian Tribes of the United States*. 6 volumes. Philadelphia: Lippincott, Grambo, and Company, 1851–1857.
Schuster, Helen H. "Yakima Indian Traditionalism: A Study in Continuity and Change." PhD diss., University of Washington, 1975.
Secretary of War, Reports of Explorations and Surveys to Ascertain the Most Practicable and Economical Route for a Railroad from the Mississippi River to the Pacific Ocean,

Made Under the Direction of the Secretary of War, in 1853–55. 12 Volumes. Washington, D.C.: Government Printing Office, 1855–1860.
Sharkey, Margery. "Revitalization and Change: A History of the Wanapum Indians, Their Prophet Smowhala, and the Washani Religion." Master's thesis, Washington State University, 1984.
Sohappy v. Smith. 302 F.Supp. 899 (D.Or. 1969).
Sprague, Roderick. "Aboriginal Burial Practices in the Plateau Region of North America." PhD diss., University of Arizona, 1967.
Stevens, Hazard. *The Life of Issac Ingalls Stevens.* 2 volumes. Boston: Houghton, Mifflin and Company, 1901.
Stewart, W. M. "David Thompson's Surveys in the North-West." *Canadian Historical Review* 17 (1936): 289–303.
Stuart, Paul. *Nations within a Nation: Historical Statistics of American Indians.* New York: Greenwood Press, 1987.
———. "The Indian Office: Growth and Development of an American Institution, 1865–1900." In *Studies in American History and Culture.* No. 12. Ann Arbor: UMI Research Press, 1979.
Trafzer, Clifford E. *Grandmother, Grandfather, and Old Wolf.* East Lansing: Michigan State University Press, 1997.
"Tuberculosis." *Med Facts.* Denver: National Jewish Center for Immunology and Respiratory Medicine, 1987.
"Tuberculosis among the North American Indians." *Report of a Committee of the National Tuberculosis Association Appointed on October 28, 1921 on Tuberculosis among the North American Indians.* Washington, D.C.: Government Printing Office, 1923.
Uncommon Controversy. A Report Prepared for the American Friends Service Committee. Seattle: University of Washington Press, 1970.
United States Bureau of Census. Census, Ninth through Fourteenth, 1870–1920.
———. *Census of Population: 1950. Characteristics of the Population, United States Summary 12,* pt. 1. Washington, D.C.: Government Printing Office, 1953.
———. *Census of Population: 1950. Special Reports. Non-white Population by Race. P-E No. 3B.* Washington, D.C.: Government Printing Office, 1953.
———. *Census of Population: 1960. Characteristics of the Population, United States Summary 1,* pt. 1. Washington. D.C.: Government Printing Office, 1964.
———. *Census of Population: 1960. Special Reports. Non-white Population by Race.* Final Report PC [2]-1C. Washington, D.C.: Government Printing Office, 1963.
———. *Report on Indians Taxed and Indians Not Taxed in the United States (Excluding Alaska) at the Eleventh Census: 1890.* Washington, D.C.: Government Printing Office, 1894.
———. *The Indian Population of the United States and Alaska: 1930.* Washington D.C.: Government Printing Office, 1930.
United States Commissioners of Indian Affairs. *Annual Reports.* 1824–1949. Reprinted by Microcard Editions, Washington, D.C., 1968.
United States Congress, House of Representatives, Committee on Interior and Insular Affairs. *Investigation of the Bureau of Indian Affairs.* 82nd Congress, 2nd Session,

House Reports, No. 2503, SS 11582. Washington, D.C.: Government Printing Office, 1953.
United States Department of the Army. *Review Report on Columbia River and Tributaries.* North Pacific Division Corps of Engineers, 1948.
United States Department of Commerce. *Historical Statistics of the United States: Colonial Times to 1970.* Washington, D.C.: Department of Commerce, 1975.
———. *The Social and Economic Status of the Black Population in the United States. An Historical View, 1790–1978.* Washington, D.C.: Department of Commerce, 1978.
United States Department of Health and Human Services. *Trends and Current Status in Childhood Mortality: United States, 1900–1985.* Washington, D.C.: Public Health Service, Center for Disease Control, 1985.
United States Department of Interior. "The Columbia River." *House Executive Document 473*, 81st Congress, 2nd Session, 1950.
———. *The Indian Population of the United States and Alaska.* Washington, D.C.: Government Printing Office, 1917.
United States Indian Health Service. *Chart Series Book, April 1986.* Washington, D.C.: Government Printing Office, 1986.
United States Public Health Service. *Whooping Cough.* Washington, D.C.: Public Health Service, 1957.
United States v. Washington. 384 F.Supp. 312 (W.D. Wash. 1974).
Washington Territorial Census, 1871. National Archives. Microfilm 276, Reel 8.
Winthrop Theodore. *The Canoe and the Saddle or Klalam and Klickitat.* Tacoma, Wash.: John H. Williams, 1913.
Yakima Tribal Council. *The Yakimas: Treaty Centennial, 1855–1955.* Yakima, Wash.: Republic Press, 1955.

Oral Interviews, Correspondence, Video

"Everything Changing, Everything Changing," Video of Ida Nason, University of Washington.
Firth, Lisa. Communication with Clifford E. Trafzer, December 1, 1992.
Francis, Lee. Communication with Clifford E. Trafzer, Bureau of Indian Affairs, April 3, 1994.
George, Andrew. Communication with Clifford E. Trafzer, May 29, 1987.
———. Communication with Clifford E. Trafzer, Richard D. Scheuerman, and Lee Ann Smith, Yakama Indian Reservation, November 15, 1981.
Guie, Geraldine. Communication with Richard D. Scheuerman, Yakima, Wash., 1983.
Holm, Kirsten. Communication with Clifford E. Trafzer, Washington Center for Health Research, April 3, 1994.
Hunn, Eugene S. Communication with Clifford E. Trafzer, May 18, 1994.
Jim, Mary. Communication with Clifford E. Trafzer and Richard D. Scheuerman, Yakama Indian Reservation, May 1, 1977; April 2 and November 10, 17, 1979; April 25, 1980.

Leslie, Craig. Photograph of Andrew George leading a Washani Funeral, Portland, Ore.
Moran, John, M.D. Communication with Clifford E. Trafzer, Yakama Indian Reservation, May 4, 1993,
Nel, Mary. Communication with Clifford E. Trafzer, Olympia, Wash., 1988.
Peone, Emily. Communication with Richard D. Scheuerman, Colville Indian Reservation, January–May, 1981.
Richie, Brad, M.D. Communication with Clifford E. Trafzer, Colton, Calif., May 18, 1993.
Sandos, James. Communication with Clifford E. Trafzer, Redlands, Calif., April 4, May 22, 1995.
Weeks, John R. Communication with Clifford E. Trafzer, June 15, 1994.

Newspapers

Los Angeles Times, May 7–8, 1995.
San Bernardino Sun, March 15, 1994.
Spokesman Review, Spokane, Washington, August 13, 1936.

Books

Armstrong, A. N. *Oregon: Comprising a Brief History and Full Descriptions of the Territories of Oregon and Washington*. Chicago: C. Scott and Company, 1857.
Bakeless, John. *Lewis and Clark, Partners in Discovery*. New York: W. Morrow, 1947.
Ballou, Robert. *Early Klickitat Valley Days*. Goldendale, Wash.: Goldendale Sentinel, 1938.
Bancroft, Hubert Howe. *History of the Northwest Coast*. San Francisco: A. L. Bancroft and Company. 1884.
———. *History of Oregon*. San Francisco: History Company, 1888.
———. *History of Washington, Idaho and Montana*. San Francisco: History Company, 1890.
———. *Native Races of the Pacific States of North America*. San Francisco: History Company, 1886.
Barnett, Homer G. *Indian Shakers: A Messianic Cult of the Pacific Northwest*. Carbondale: Southern Illinois University Press, 1972.
Bates, Barbara. *Bargaining for Life: A Social History of Tuberculosis, 1876–1938*. Philadelphia: University of Pennsylvania Press, 1992.
Beavert, Virginia, ed. *The Way It Was: Anaku Iwacha*. Toppenish, Wash.: Franklin Press, 1974.
Berreman, Joel V. *Tribal Distribution in Oregon*. Menasha, Wis.: American Anthropological Association, 1937.
Brown, William J., James F. Donohue, Norman W. Axnick, Joseph H. Blount, Neal H. Ewen, and Oscar G. Jones. *Syphilis and Other Venereal Diseases*. Cambridge: Harvard University Press, 1970.

Buikstra, Jane E., ed. *Prehistoric Tuberculosis in the Americas*. Scientific Papers, no. 5. Evanston, Illinois: Northwestern University Archaeological Program, 1981.
Burnet, Frank MacFarlan, and David O. White. *Natural History of Infectious Diseases*. Cambridge: Cambridge University Press, 1972.
Burns, Robert Ignatius. *The Jesuits and the Indian Wars of the Northwest*. New Haven: Yale University Press, 1966.
Cannon, Miles. *Waiilatpu, Its Rise and Fall, 1836–1847: A Story of Pioneer Days in the Pacific Northwest*. Boise, Idaho: Capital News Job Rooms, 1915.
Caputi, Jane. *Gossips, Gorgons & Crones: The Fates of the Earth*. Santa Fe: Bear & Company, 1993.
Cartwright, Frederick Fox. *Disease and History*. London: Hart-Davis, 1972.
Chalfant, Stuart. *Interior Salish and Eastern Washington Indians*. New York: Garland Publishing, 1974.
Christie, Andrew B. *Infectious Diseases: Epidemiology and Clinical Practice*. Edinburgh and London: E. and S. Livingstone, 1969.
Chuinard, E. G. *The Medical Aspects of the Lewis and Clark Expedition*. Corvallis, Ore.: Oregon State University Friends of the Library, 1954.
Clark, Ella. *Indian Legends of the Pacific Northwest*. Berkeley: University of California Press, 1953.
Cohen, Felix S. *Handbook of Federal Indian Law*. Albuquerque: University of New Mexico Press, 1971.
Collins, Selwyn Dewitt, and Josephine Lehmann. *Excess Deaths from Influenza and Pneumonia and from Important Chronic Diseases during Epidemic Periods, 1918–1951*. Washington, D.C.: Public Health Service, 1953.
Cook, Sherburne F. *The Conflict between the California Indian and White Civilization*. Berkeley: University of California Press, 1976.
———. *The Population of the California Indians, 1769–1970*. Berkeley: University of California Press, 1976.
———. *Population Trends among the California Mission Indians*. Ibero-Americana, no. 17. University of California Publications, 1940.
Corner, Beryl Dorothy. *Prematurity: The Diagnosis, Care and Disorders of the Premature Infant*. London: Cassell, 1960.
Crosby, Alfred W. *Ecological Imperialism: The Biological Expansion of Europe, 1900–1900*. Cambridge: Cambridge University Press, 1986.
———. *The Columbian Exchange: Biological and Cultural Consequences of 1492*. Westport, Conn.: Greenwood Publishing Company, 1972.
Culverwell, Albert. *Stronghold in the Yakima Country*. Olympia, Wash.: Washington State Parks and Recreation Commission, 1956.
Desmond, G. B. *Gambling among the Yakimas*. Washington, D.C.: Catholic University of America Press, 1952.
Dobyns, Henry F. *Native American Historical Demography: A Critical Bibliography*. Bloomington: Indiana University Press, 1976.
———. *Their Number Became Thinned: Native American Population Dynamics in Eastern North America*. Knoxville: University of Tennessee Press, 1983.
Drury, Clifford M. *Marcus Whitman*. Caldwell, Idaho: Caxton Printers, Ltd., 1936.

———. *Marcus Whitman, M.D.: Pioneer and Martyr.* Caldwell, Idaho: Caxton Printers, Ltd., 1937.
———. *Tepee in His Front Yard.* Portland, Ore.: Binfords and Mort, 1949.
Dubos, Rent, and Jean Dubos. *The White Plague: Tuberculosis, Man, and Society.* Boston: Little, Brown & Company, 1952. Reprinted in 1992 by Rutgers University Press, New Brunswick, New Jersey.
Getches, David H., and Charles F. Wilkinson. *Federal Indian Law.* St. Paul, Minn.: West Publishing Company, 1986.
Gibbs, George. *Indian Tribes of Washington Territory.* Fairfield, Wash.: Ye Galleon Press, 1972.
Gibson, Arrell M. *The American Indian: Prehistory to Present.* Lexington, Mass.: D.C. Heath, 1980.
Gidley, M. *With One Sky above Us.* Seattle: University of Washington Press, 1974.
Gilbert, Frank T. *The Whitman Massacre, with a Few Prior Historical Events.* Portland, Ore.: North Pacific History Company, 1888.
Guie, H. Dean. *Bugles in the Valley: The Story of Garnett's Fort Simcoe.* Portland: Oregon Historical Society, 1977.
Heizer, Robert F. *Handbook of North American Indians: Volume 8—California.* Washington, D.C.: Smithsonian Institution Press, 1978.
Hess, Julius H., and Evelyn C. Lundeen. *The Premature Infant.* Philadelphia: Lippincott, 1949.
Hines, Donald M. *Magic in the Mountains. The Yakima Shaman: Power and Practice.* Issaquah, Wash.: Great Eagle Publishing, 1993.
Hodge, Frederick W., ed. *Handbook of American Indians North of Mexico.* 2 volumes. Washington, D.C.: United States Government Printing Office, 1907–1910.
Hoopes, A. W. *Indian Affairs and Their Administration, 1849–1860, with Especial Reference to the Far West.* Philadelphia: University of Pennsylvania Press, 1932.
Howard, Cheryl. *Navajo Tribal Demography, 1983–1986: A Comparative and Historical Perspective.* New York: Garland, 1993.
Hrdlicka, Ales. *Tuberculosis among Certain Indian Tribes in the United States.* Annual Report of the Bureau of American Ethnography, Bulletin 42. Washington, D.C.: Smithsonian Institution, 1909.
Hull, Lindley M. *A History of Central Washington, Including the Famous Wenatchee, Entiat, Chelan and Columbia Valleys.* Spokane, Wash.: Shaw and Borden Company, 1932.
Hultkrantz, Ake. *Conceptions of the Soul among North American Indians.* Stockholm: Ethnographical Museum of Sweden, 1953.
———. *The North American Indian Orpheus Tradition.* Stockholm: Ethnographical Museum of Sweden, 1957.
Hunn, Eugene S., with James Selam. *Nch'i-Wana, "The Big River": Mid-Columbia Indians and Their Land.* Seattle: University of Washington Press, 1990.
Johansen, Dorothy O., and Charles M. Gates. *Empire of the Columbia: A History of the Pacific Northwest.* New York: Harper & Row, 1967.
Josephy, Alvin M., Jr. *The Nez Perce Indians and the Opening of the Northwest.* New Haven, Conn.: Yale University Press, 1965.

Kimmel, Thelma. *The Fort Simcoe Story*. Toppenish, Wash.: Toppenish Review, 1954.
Kuntz, Jeffrey, and Asher J. Finkle. *The American Medical Association Family Medical Guide*. New York: Random House, 1987.
Kvasnicka, Robert M., and Herman J. Viola, eds. *The Commissioners of Indian Affairs*. Lincoln: University of Nebraska Press, 1979.
La Barre, Weston. *Ghost Dance: Origins of Religion*. New York: Dell Publishing Company, 1972.
Lapin, Joseph H. *Whooping Cough*. Springfield, Ill.: C. C. Thomas, 1943.
Lebenthan, Emanuel, ed. *Textbook of Gastroenterology and Nutrition in Infancy*. New York: Raven Press, 1981.
Lundeen, Evelyn C., and Ralph H. Kunstadter. *Care of the Premature Infant*. Philadelphia: Lippincott, 1958.
Lyman, W. D. *History of the Yakima Valley, Washington, Comprising Yakima, Kittitas and Benton Counties*. Chicago: S. J. Clarke, 1919.
Lynn ,William S. *Inflammatory Cells and Lung Disease*. Boca Raton, Fla.: CRC Press, 1983.
McKeown, Thomas. *The Modern Rise of Population*. New York: Academic Press, 1976.
McNeil, William H. *Plagues and People*. Garden City, N.Y.: Anchor Doubleday, 1976.
McWhorter, Lucullus Virgil. *The Crime against the Yakima*. North Yakima, Wash.: Republic Press, 1913.
Meinig, Donald W. *The Great Columbia Plain: A Historical Geography, 1805–1910*. Seattle: University of Washington Press, 1968.
Meyers, Jay Arthur. *Captains of All These Men of Death*. St. Louis, Miss.: Warren H. Green, 1977.
Miller, Jay, ed. *Mourning Dove: A Salishan Autobiography*. Lincoln: University of Nebraska Press, 1990.
Moyers, Bill, ed. *Healing and the Mind*. New York: Doubleday, 1993.
Nash, Gary. *Red, White, and Black: The Peoples of Early America*. Englewood Cliffs, N.J.: Prentice-Hall, 1974.
Nashone. *Grandmother Stories of the Northwest*. Newcastle, Calif.: Sierra Oaks Publishing Company, 1987.
Newell, Colin. *Methods and Models in Demography*. London: Belhaven Press, 1988.
Oliphant, J. Orin. *On the Cattle Ranges of the Oregon Country*. Seattle: University of Washington Press, 1968.
Oregon Improvement Company. *Eastern Washington Territory and Oregon*. Portland: Oregon Improvement Company, 1881.
Ortiz, Alfonso, ed. *Handbook of North American Indians Southwest*. Washington, D.C.: Smithsonian Institution Press, 1983.
Pennington, James E., ed. *Respiratory Infections: Diagnosis and Management*. New York: Raven Press, 1983.
Philp, Kenneth R. *John Collier's Crusade for Indian Reform, 1920–1954*. Tucson: University of Arizona Press, 1972.
Preston, Samuel, and Michael R. Haines. *Fatal Years: Child Mortality in Late Nineteenth Century America*. Princeton: Princeton University Press, 1991.

Prucha, Francis Paul. *American Indian Policy in Crisis: Christian Reformers and the Indian, 1865–1900.* Norman: University of Oklahoma Press, 1976.

———. *Indian Policy in the United States.* Lincoln: University of Nebraska Press, 1981.

Ramenofsky, Ann F. *Vectors of Death.* Albuquerque: University of New Mexico Press, 1987.

Ray, Verne F. *Cultural Relations in the Plateau of Northwestern America.* Los Angeles: Southwest Museum, 1939.

Reichwein, Jeffrey C. *Emergence of Native American Nationalism in the Columbia Plateau.* New York: Garland Publishing Company, 1990.

Relander, Click. *Drummers and Dreamers.* Caldwell, Idaho: Caxton Printers, Ltd., 1956.

———. *Strangers on the Land.* Yakima, Wash.: Franklin Press, 1962.

———. *The Yakimas: Treaty Centennial.* Yakima, Wash.: Republic Press, 1955.

Richards, Kent. *Isaac L. Stevens: Young Man in a Hurry.* Provo, Utah: Brigham Young University Press, 1979. Reprinted by Washington State University Press, 1993.

Rollins, Phillip A., ed. *The Discovery of the Oregon Trail.* New York: Charles Scribner's Sons, 1935.

Ronda, James P. *Lewis and Clark among the Indians.* Lincoln: University of Nebraska Press, 1984.

Ruby, Robert H., and John A. Brown. *The Cayuse Indians: Imperial Tribesmen of Old Oregon.* Norman: University of Oklahoma Press, 1972.

———. *Dreamer-Prophets of the Columbia Plateau: Smohalla and Skolaskin.* Norman: University of Oklahoma Press, 1989.

———. *A Guide to the Indian Tribes of the Pacific Northwest.* Norman: University of Oklahoma Press, 1986.

———. *Indians of the Pacific Northwest.* Norman: University of Oklahoma Press, 1982.

———. *John Slocum and the Indian Shaker Church.* Norman: University of Oklahoma Press, 1996.

Schuster, Helen H. *The Yakima.* Indians of North America Series, ed. Frank W. Porter III. New York: Chelsea House Publishers, 1990.

———. *The Yakimas: A Critical Bibliography.* Bloomington: Indiana University Press, 1982.

Shryock, Henry S., Jacob S. Siegel, and Associates, with condensed edition by Edward G. Stockwell. *The Methods and Materials of Demography.* San Diego: Academic Press, 1976.

Shryock, Richard Harrison. *National Tuberculosis Association, 1904–1954.* New York: National Tuberculosis Association, 1957.

Simpson, Howard. *Invisible Armies.* Indianapolis: Bobbs-Merrill, 1980.

Sleisenger, Marvin H., and John S. Fordham, eds. *Gastrointestinal Disease.* Philadelphia: W. B. Saunders, 1989.

Smith, F. B. *The Retreat of Tuberculosis, 1850–1950.* London: Croom Helm, 1988.

Snipp, C. M. *American Indians: The First of this Land.* New York: Russell-Sage Foundation, 1987.

Spier, Leslie. *The Prophet Dance of the Northwest and Its Derivatives: The Source of the Ghost Dance.* General Series in Anthropology. Menasha, Wis.: George Banta Publishing Co., 1953.

———. *Tribal Distribution in Washington.* General Series in Anthropology. Menasha, Wis.: George Banta Publishing Co., 1936.

Spink, Wesley W. *Infectious Diseases: Prevention and Treatment in the Nineteenth and Twentieth Centuries.* Minneapolis: University of Minnesota Press, 1978.

Splawn, A. J. *Ka-mi-akin, Last Hero of the Yakimas.* Portland, Ore.: Stationary and Printing Company, 1917.

Stearn, E. Wagner, and Allen E. Stearn. *The Effect of Smallpox on the Destiny of the Amerindian.* Boston: Bruce Humphries, Inc., 1945.

Swanton, John R. *Indian Tribes of North America.* Washington, D.C.: Government Printing Office, 1952.

Teller, Michael. *The Tuberculosis Movement: A Public Health Campaign in the Progressive Era.* New York: Greenwood Press, 1988.

Thornton, Russell. *American Indian Holocaust and Survival: A Population History since 1492.* Norman: University of Oklahoma Press, 1978.

Trafzer, Clifford E., ed. *American Indian Identity: Today's Changing Perspectives.* Newcastle, Calif.: Sierra Oaks Publishing Co., 1989.

———. *American Indian Prophets.* Newcastle, Calif.: Sierra Oaks Publishing Co., 1986.

———. *Chief Joseph's Allies.* Newcastle, Calif.: Sierra Oaks Publishing Company, 1992.

———. *The Chinook.* New York: Chelsea House Publishers, 1990.

———. *Death Stalks the Yakama: Epidemiological Transitions and Mortality on the Yakama Indian Reservation, 1888–1964.* East Lansing: Michigan State University Press, 1997.

———. *Indians, Superintendents, and Councils: Northwestern Indian Policy, 1850–1855.* Lanham, Md.: University Press of America, 1986.

———. *Yakima, Palouse, Cayuse, Umatilla, Walla Walla, and Wanapum: An Historical Bibliography.* Metuchen, N.J.: Scarecrow Press, 1992.

Trafzer, Clifford E., and Richard D. Scheuerman. *Renegade Tribe: The Palouse Indians and the Invasion of the Inland Pacific Northwest.* Pullman: Washington University Press, 1986.

Trevanthan, Wenda R. *Human Birth: An Evolutionary Perspective.* New York: Aldine Le Gruyter, 1987.

Truelove, S. C. *Diseases of the Digestive System.* Oxford: Blackwell Scientific Publications, 1972.

Tyler, Lyman. *A History of Indian Policy.* Washington, D.C.: Government Printing Office, 1973.

Villard, Henry. *The Early History of Transportation in Oregon.* Eugene: University of Oregon Press, 1944.

Vogel, Virgil J. *American Indian Medicine.* Norman: University of Oklahoma Press, 1970.

Waksman, Selman A. *The Conquest of Tuberculosis.* Berkeley: University of California Press, 1964.

Weeks, John R. *Population: An Introduction to Concepts and Issues.* Belmont, Calif.: Wadsworth Publishing Company, 1992.

Williams, J. D., and J. Burnie, eds. *Bacterial Meningitis.* London: Academic Press, 1987.

Zucker, Jeff, Kay Hummel, and Bob Hogfoss. *Oregon Indians: Culture, History, and Current Affairs, An Atlas and Introduction.* Portland: Oregon Historical Society, 1983.

Articles and Chapters

Alter, George. "Infant and Child Mortality in the United States and Canada." Paper presented at "La Mortalite des Enfants dans le Passé" conference, International Union for the Scientific Study of Population, October 7–9, 1992.

Basso, Keith H. "Western Apache." *Handbook of North American Indians Southwest.* Washington, D.C.: Smithsonian Institution Press, 1983.

Bischoff, William N. "Yakima Campaign of 1856." *Mid-America* 31 (1949): 163–208.

———. "The Yakima Indian War, 1855–56, A Problem in Research." *Pacific Northwest Quarterly* 41 (1950): 162–69.

Bosch, F. Xavier, et al. "Male Sexual Behavior and Human Papilloma Virus DNA: Key Risk Factors for Cervical Cancer in Spain." *Journal of the National Cancer Institute* 88 (1996): 1060–75.

Boyd, Robert T. "Pacific Northwest Measles Epidemic, 1847–1848." *Oregon Historical Quarterly* 95 (1994): 6–47.

Buechner, Helmutt K. "Some Biotic Changes in the State of Washington, Particularly during the Century 1853–1953." *Research Studies of the State College of Washington* 21 (1953): 154–92.

Campbell, Gregory R. "The Changing Dimensions of Native American Health: A Critical Understanding of Contemporary Native American Health Issues." *American Indian Culture and Research Journal* 13 (1989): 1–20.

———. "The Political Epidemiology of Infant Mortality: A Crisis among Montana American Indians." *American Indian Culture and Research Journal* 13 (1989): 105–48.

Carmichael, Ann G. "Infection, Hidden Hunger, and History." *Journal of Interdisciplinary History* 14 (1983): 249–64.

Carr, Barbara A., and Eun Sul Lee. "Navajo Tribal Mortality: A Life Table Analysis of the Leading Cause of Death." *Social Biology* 25 (1978): 279–87.

Castillo, Edward D. "The Impact of Euro-American Exploration and Settlement." *Handbook of North American Indians California*, ed. Robert F. Heizer, 99–127. Washington, D.C.: Smithsonian Institution Press, 1978.

Clark, Ella. "George Gibbs' Account of Indian Mythology in Oregon and Washington Territories." *Oregon Historical Quarterly* 56 (1955–1956): 293–325, and 57 (1955–1956): 125–67.

Coale, George L. "Notes on the Guardian Spirit Concept Among the Nez Perce." *National Archives of Ethnography* 48 (1958).

Coan, C. F. "The Adoption of the Reservation Policy in the Pacific Northwest, 1853–1855." *Oregon Historical Quarterly* 23 (1922): 1–38.

———. "The First Stage of the Federal Indian Policy in the Pacific Northwest." *Oregon Historical Quarterly* 22 (1921): 46–89.

Colton, J. S. "A Report on the Range Conditions of Central Washington." *Washington State Agricultural College Experiment Station Bulletin* 60 (1904): 5–21.

Cook, Shelburne F. "The Epidemic of 1830–33 in California and Oregon." *University of California Publications in American Archaeology and Ethnology* 43 (1955): 303–26.

Culverwell, Albert. "Stronghold in the Yakima Country: Fort Simcoe and the Indian War, 1856–59." *Pacific Northwest Quarterly* 46 (1955): 46–51.

DeLien, H., and J. Nixon Hadley. "How to Recognize an Indian Health Problem." *Human Organization* (1952): 29–33.

Deutsch, Herman J. "Indian and White in the Inland Empire: The Contest for the Land, 1880–1912." *Pacific Northwest Quarterly* 47 (1956): 44–51.

Dickinson, John A. "The Pre-Contact Huron Population: A Reappraisal." *Ontario History* 72 (1980): 173–79.

Dobyns, Henry F. "Estimating Aboriginal American Population: An Appraisal of Techniques with a New Hemisphere Estimate." *Current Anthropology* 7 (1966): 395–416.

———. *Tribalism Today: An Anthropological Perspective on Reservation Enclaves and Urban Pan-Indians.*" Paper presented at First Annual Conference on Problems and Issues Concerning American Indians Today, Newberry Library, 1978.

Douglas, Jesse S. "Origins of the Population in Oregon in 1850." *Pacific Northwest Quarterly* 41 (1950): 95–108.

Emerson, Haven. "Morbidity of the American Indians." *Science* 63 (1926): 229–31.

Hadley J. Nixon. "Demography of the American Indians." *Annals of the American Academy of Political and Social Science* 311 (1957): 23–30.

Haines, Francis. "The Northward Spread of Horses among the Plains Indians." *American Anthropologist* 40 (1938): 429–37.

———. "Problems of Indian Policy." *Pacific Northwest Quarterly* 41 (1950): 203–12.

Hilgard, E. W. "The Yakima and the Clickitat Regions." *The Northwest* 2 (1884): 1–12.

Hill, Charles A., Jr., and Mozart I. Spector. "Natality and Mortality of American Indians Compared with United States Whites and Nonwhites." *Health Reports* 86 (1971): 229–46.

Hoaglin, Lester L., Jr., and Herbert C. Taylor Jr. "The Intermittent Fever Epidemic of the 1830's on the Lower Columbia River." *Ethnohistory* 2 (1962): 160–78.

Jacobs, Melville. "A Sketch of Northern Sahaptin Grammar." *University of Washington Publications in Anthropology* 4 (1931): 83–292.

Johansson, S. Ryan. "Food For Thought: Rhetoric and Reality in Modern Mortality History." *Historical Methods* 27 (1994): 101–25.

Joralemon, Donald. "New World Depopulation and the Case of Disease." *Journal of Anthropological Research* 38 (1982): 108–27.

Justice, James W. "Twenty Years of Diabetes on the Warm Springs Reservation, Oregon." *American Indian Culture and Research Journal* 13 (1989): 49–81.

Konlande, J. R., and J. R. K. Robson. "The Nutritive Value of Cooked Camas as Consumed by Flathead Indians." *Ecology of Food and Nutrition* 2 (1972): 193–95.
Lee, M. R. Roburn, and A. Carrow. "Nutritional Studies of British Columbian Indians." *Canadian Journal of Public Health* 62 (1971): 285–96.
McKeown, Thomas. "Food, Infection, and Population." *Journal of Interdisciplinary History* 14 (1983): 227–47.
Morse, Dan. "Prehistoric Tuberculosis in America." *American Review of Respiratory Diseases* 83 (1961): 489–504.
Neel, James V. "Diabetes Mellitus: A 'Thrifty' Genotype Rendered Detrimental by 'Progress.'" *American Journal of Human Genetics* 14 (1962): 353–62.
Nelson, Denys. "Yakima Days." *Washington Historical Quarterly* 19 (1928): 45–51, 117–33, 181–92.
Newman, Marshall T. "Aboriginal New World Epidemiology and Medical Care, and the Impact of the Old World Disease Imports." *American Journal of Physical Anthropology* 45 (1976): 667–72.
Norton, Helen J., and Steven J. Gill. "The Ethnobotanical Imperative: A Consideration of Obligations, Implications, and Methodology." *Northwest Anthropological Research Notes* 15 (1981): 117–87.
Oliphant, J. Orin. "Encroachment of Cattlemen on Indian Reservations in the Pacific Northwest, 1870–1890." *Agricultural History* 24 (1950): 42–58.
———. "Some Neglected Aspects of the History of the Pacific Northwest." *Pacific Northwest Quarterly* 61 (1970): 1–9.
Omran, Abdel R. "Epidemiologic Transition in the United States: The Health Factor in Population Change." *Population Bulletin* 32 (1977): 1–42.
Painter, Harry. "New Light on Chief Kamiakin." *Walla Walla Union Bulletin*, March 18, 1945.
Popkin, Barry M. "Nutritional Patterns and Transitions." *Population and Development Review* 19 (1993): 138–57.
Raviglione, Mario, Dixie Snider, and Arata Kochi. "Global Epidemiology of Tuberculosis." *Journal of the American Medical Association* 18 (1995): 220–26.
Ray, Verne E. "The Bluejay Character in the Plateau Spirit Dance." *American Anthropologist* 39 (1937): 593–601.
———. "Native Villages and Groupings of the Columbia Basin." *Pacific Northwest Quarterly* 27 (1936): 99–152.
———. "Tribal Distribution in Eastern Oregon and Adjacent Regions." *American Anthropologist* 40 (1938): 384–415.
Richards, Kent. "Issac Stevens and Federal Military Power in Washington Territory." *Pacific Northwest Quarterly* 63 (1972): 81–86.
Rosen, Laurence S., and Kurt Gorwitz. "New Attention to American Indians." *American Demographics* 2 (1980): 18–25.
Roth, Eric Abella. "Demography and Computer Simulation in Historic Village Population Reconstruction." *Journal of Anthropological Research* 3 (1981): 279–301.
Schneider, Keith. "Nuclear Complex Threatens Indians." *New York Times*, National Edition, September 3, 1990.

Scott, Leslie M. "Indian Disease as Aids to Pacific Northwest Settlement." *Oregon Historical Quarterly* 19 (1928): 99–107.

Siegel, Jacob S. "Estimates of Coverage of the Population by Sex, Race, and Age in the 1970 Census." *Demography* 11 (1974): 1–23.

Slagle, Al Logan. "Tolowa Indian Shakers and the Role of Prophecy at Smith River, California." In *American Indian Prophets*, ed. Clifford E. Trafzer. Newcastle, Calif.: Sierra Oaks Publishing Company, 1981.

Stanley, Sam, and Robert K. Thomas. "Current Demographic and Social Trends among North American Indians." *Annals of the American Academy of Political and Social Science* 436 (1978): 111–20.

Stearn, E. Wagner, and Allen E. Stearn. "Smallpox Immunization of the Amerindian." *Bulletin of the History of Medicine* 13 (1943): 601–13.

Taylor, Herbert C., Jr., and Lester L. Hoaglin. "The 'Intermittent Fever.' Epidemic of the 1830s on the Lower Columbia River." *Ethnohistory* 9 (1962): 160–78.

Thornton, Russell. "American Indian Historical Demography: A Review Essay with Suggestions for Future Research." *American Indian Culture and Research Journal* 3 (1979): 69–74.

Thornton, Russell, and Joan Marsh-Thornton. "Estimating Prehistoric American Indian Population Size for United States Area: Implications of the Nineteenth Century Population Decline and Nadir." *American Journal of Physical Anthropology* 55 (1981): 47–53.

Trafzer, Clifford E. "Horses, Cattle, Buggies, Hacks: Purchases by Yakima Indian Women, 1909–1912." In *Negotiators of Change: Historical Perspectives on Native American Women*, ed. Nancy Shoemaker, 176–92. New York: Routledge, 1995.

Trafzer, Clifford E., and Margery Ann Beach. "Smohalla, the Washani, and Religion as a Factor in Northwestern Indian History." *American Indian Quarterly* 9 (1985): 309–24.

Wagner, Carruth J., and Erwin S. Rabeau. "Indian Poverty and Indian Health." *United States Department of Health, Education, and Welfare Indicators* (1964): xxiv–xliv.

Watkins, Susan Cott, and Etienne van de Walle. "Nutrition, Mortality, and Population Size: Malthus' Court of Last Resort." *Journal of Interdisciplinary History* 14 (1983): 205–26.

Weiss, K. M., and P. E. Smouse. "The Demographic Stability of Small Human Populations." In *The Demographic Evolution of Human Populations*. London: Academic Press, 1976.

Whitner, R. L. "Grant's Indian Peace Policy on the Yakima Reservation, 1870–1882." *Pacific Northwest Quarterly* 50 (1959): 135–42.

Index

Note: Italic numbers refer to tables.

www.ingramcontent.com/pod-product-compliance
Ingram Content Group UK Ltd.
Pitfield, Milton Keynes, MK11 3LW, UK
UKHW041629031026
15587UKWH00001B/161

9 780810 866478